Contents

Introduction

The number of people diagnosed with diabetes all over the world has grown to an incredible degree in recent years, making it a growing concern for governments and health services alike. This condition is not a disease - you don't catch it, you develop it. At present, there is a minimum of 2 million people in the UK living with diabetes, but it's also estimated that up to 1 million may have the condition without realising.

There are a number of different factors that can trigger the development of diabetes, but there are two major causes which allow us to distinguish between the two main forms of diabetes: Type 1, or insulin-dependent, and Type 2, non-insulin-dependent. Of the 2 million we do know about, about one quarter have Type 1 diabetes, while the remainder have Type 2. While both types of diabetes can be treated with insulin, those with Type 2 can also produce a certain amount of insulin themselves.

At one point, Type 2 diabetes was considered a condition only adults could have. However, the number of children and adolescents with this type of diabetes is now also skyrocketing. The number of Type 2 diabetes cases in children from Japan has doubled over the last two decades, making it more common than Type 1. In the US, it's estimated that between 8-45% of new diabetes cases in children are of Type 2 diabetes. Only 1.3-5.3% of aboriginal and native children from Australia and North America have been diagnosed with Type 2 diabetes.

While this is a condition which should be taken seriously, it's important to understand that it's entirely possible to have a regular, balanced life while dealing with it. You just need some helpful advice, an understanding of how your blood sugars are impacted by your diet, and a good amount of discipline. This book hopes to provide as much relevant medical information and practical advice as possible.

We'll explore what diabetes is and how a person develops it, how they can live a full, healthy life with the condition, what treatments are available. For further information, there's also a glossary of all the most important words at the back of the book. Whether you know someone with diabetes or have just been diagnosed yourself, this book will give you all the tips you need.

A Note to the Reader

This book provides general information on diabetes, but should not be used in the place of professional medical advice. It can be a very helpful guide to use alongside your doctor's advice. If you have any concerns about your condition or whether or not you may have diabetes, please talk to your healthcare provider. While every care has been taken to ensure that the information in this text is accurate, the author does not claim to have the proper qualifications to diagnose this condition.

Please talk to your doctor before undertaking any form of treatment.

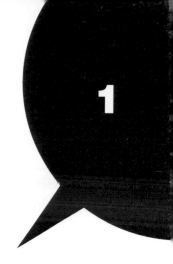

1

What is Diabetes? (Types, Symptoms and Diagnoses)

Diabetes is a condition in which your body is unable to regulate its blood sugar on its own. Doctors will diagnose you with this condition on reading your blood sugar levels if the result is too high. Usually, 'too high' is anywhere over eight millimoles per litre (mmols/L).

How is blood sugar controlled in non-diabetics?

In those who don't have diabetes, this happens by a feedback mechanism.

1. The person eats something.

2. As the food is digested, blood sugar levels begin to rise.

3. The pituitary gland in the person's brain reads the sugar level in the blood that reaches it.

4. If the level is higher than it should be, the gland sends a message through the blood to the pancreas, causing it to produce insulin. This lowers the blood sugar level.

5. If the level is lower than it should be, the gland sends a message to the liver which then releases energy as glucagon. This raises the blood sugar level.

6. The pituitary gland continues to release these messengers until the blood sugar level is balanced.

Symptoms of Diabetes

The most common symptoms for diabetes include…

- Increased thirstiness
- Extreme tiredness
- Blurred vision
- Weight loss
- Needing to urinate unusually often, especially at night

The two main types of diabetes are Type 1 and Type 2. As a general rule, Type 1 diabetes will develop more quickly than Type 2, usually over a number of weeks, with very obvious symptoms. Meanwhile, Type 2 diabetes will develop more gradually, and its symptoms are normally less extreme. In some cases, those with this condition won't realise they have it at all until it's spotted in a medical check-up.

Some people with Type 2 diabetes mistake their symptoms for signs that they're simply overworking or ageing. With both types of diabetes, these symptoms will improve rapidly as soon as treatment begins. Treating the condition early on also reduces the chances of patients developing more serious health problems, which can be caused by untreated diabetes.

Diabetes in the Workplace: Information for Employers

The Department of Health states that up to 21% of the UK population is clinically obese, which costs more than £2 billion in lost productivity each year (due to 18 million sick days). It's highly likely that around 4% of your employees will have diabetes.

Hints and Advice

- It's reasonable to expect that someone with diabetes will include this information on a job application if you provide a section for disabilities and illnesses.

- Talk to your employee to get a better idea of how they think their condition might affect their ability to carry out their job. In most cases, all this will amount to is a need for occasional extra snacks to raise blood sugar, and blood tests from time to time.

- If your employee appears to need help, there's nothing wrong with offering it. For example, it can be helpful to know where there is sugar in the event of a hypoglycaemic episode.

- If your employee has a hypo, they may not have any reason to tell you about it. However, it can take around 15 minutes to recover from these episodes, so you should allow them this time if they ask for it.

- Diabetes should never be considered to be a reason not to employ someone.

What happens in a diabetic?

Type 1 diabetes

Type 1 diabetes is caused by a genetic component which means the person isn't able to produce any insulin themselves. In the past, this was the only type of diabetes that children would be diagnosed with, so it was often called juvenile diabetes.

In some cases, children with Type 1 diabetes are only given one type of insulin, while others may need to take two. The condition will require one or two injections each day, but can sometimes take even more than that. We will discuss changes in insulin treatments as a child grows later in the book.

Contrary to popular belief, you can't develop Type 1 diabetes simply as a result of having a bad diet. Type 1 diabetes occurs when your immune system mistakes beta cells - which produce insulin and are found in the islets of Langerhans in the pancreas - as a foreign body, and destroying them as a result. The only link between this condition and the food you eat is that you'll have a heightened awareness of how different foods affect your health, with sugary foods having a very noticeable effect.

We have not yet worked out how to predict who will and won't develop this conditions, but it is clear that those who have ancestors with the condition are more likely to develop it. Once you're diagnosed with diabetes, you'll have to keep track of the food you eat, especially thecarbohydrates, and do frequent blood tests so that you know how much insulin you need to balance out what you eat. This will be done either by injection or by insulin pump.

Please note also that your body needs insulin no matter what you eat. If you're unwell and aren't eating, you still need to take your insulin in order to survive. Similarly, if you decide to lose weight by eating less, this won't mean you get to stop taking insulin. Reduce the amount of insulin you take in order to match your new food intake, but don't stop taking it altogether.

> If you're unwell and aren't eating, you still need to take your insulin in order to survive. Similarly, if you decide to lose weight by eating less, this won't mean you get to stop taking insulin. Reduce the amount of insulin you take in order to match your new food intake, but don't stop taking it altogether.

Type 2 diabetes

Type 2 diabetes is the diagnosis given to those who can make their own insulin to a certain extent, but whose insulin is less effective than normal. This condition can stem from exercising too little, being overweight or eating an unhealthy diet. Some experts believe that Type 2 diabetes is becoming worryingly common in our times as a result of certain societal changes, such as supermarkets, the replacement of walking with driving and the increased access to fast foods.

Although there are certain genetic and medical factors (the 'fat gene,' for example) which can contribute to such weight gain, around 80% of those with Type 2 diabetes have excess weight and eat a bad diet. Following your initial diagnosis with Type 2 diabetes, it's likely your diet will be reviewed and your blood sugar levels stabilised by pills. You may not be given insulin at first, but this may still occur later in treatment.

Gestational Diabetes

This is a condition which affects around 4% of all pregnant people. Good diabetes management is extra-important here, as unhealthy blood sugar levels can be bad for your unborn child. In order to look after your bump, you'll need to look after yourself through careful diet and frequent blood tests. Distinct from Type 1 and Type 2, gestational diabetes appears when someone is pregnant and then disappears after they give birth.

People with this condition generally need to control their diabetes in similar ways to those with long-term diabetes, though in many cases treatment will only involve diet and pills rather than insulin. In cases where the diabetes continues after the birth of your baby, you will then be diagnosed with either Type 1 or Type 2, meaning that you may have already had diabetes which only became apparent when you became pregnant.

Working Out Dosages

For those with Type 1 diabetes, blood tests must be done to measure the blood sugar level. Once this is assessed, it's a matter of doing the necessary maths to plan your dosage. The factors to take into account here are…

- **Blood sugar.** It's best to test your blood sugar level before eating a meal
- **Activities.** What are you planning to do after eating? How much energy will you require?
- **Meal.** What food are you about to eat?

Because every body is different, there isn't a specific formula for working out your dosage. It all comes down to time, judgement, perseverance, continual monitoring and practice. You won't always be able to have the perfect level of blood sugar, but you will learn over time how to predict how your body will react to the food you eat.

One basic guideline you may like to follow is to take a unit of insulin for each 10g of carbohydrate you consume. This is why some people refer to 10g of carbohydrate as 'one exchange'. There are a few factors which will determine how much insulin you need to give yourself...

- Which type of insulin do you take? How does it work?
- What are you about to eat? How many carbohydrates are in the dish?
- What are you going to do after eating? (If you're about to expend a lot of energy, you'll need less insulin than if you're going to be sitting around).
- What is your body size?

One of the biggest learning curves you'll encounter when you're first diagnosed with diabetes is counting your carbohydrates. This is something that can take a while to get used to, but in time it'll become second nature. If you've ever been on a diet which has required you to count calories, this is something similar.

We'll talk more about counting carbohydrates later in the book.

Blood tests: What, How and Why?

Diabetes is characterised by above-average blood sugar levels, which can generally be moderated through the use of medication. High blood sugars can damage the body over time. Diabetes diagnoses are based on a number of blood test results which show unusually high blood sugar readings. It's possible you will need blood tests on a daily basis after your diagnosis to stay on top of what's happening in your body.

To carry out a blood test, you'll need...

- A blood test machine.
- A lancing device.
- A sensor (or blood test strip).

It can also be a good idea to keep a blood glucose diary to keep track of your results.

Blood Test Strips

Blood test strips (also known as blood test sensors or electrodes) can be attained for free with a prescription from your GP following a diabetes diagnosis. However, in order to access them for free you may need to discuss how many strips you're likely to need on a weekly or monthly basis based on your blood testing regime, and you may need to get a Medical Exemption Certificate.

For example, if you test your blood five times each day, you'll need 35 strips per week. Strips generally come in tubs of around 20, so you may need to get more than one tub each week. Your doctor is likely to also carry out a HbA1c test.

The HbA1c Blood Test

This is a blood test which will be carried out specifically by your doctor or nurse, and which has come to be seen as a sort of *Holy Grail* for diabetics. The number you get in your results will be something you really need to think about as it's a very strong indication of how likely you are to develop complications as a result of your diabetes. Unless your doctor has the relevant blood test machine for this test, you may need to wait a week or two for your results, but it'll be worth it.

The result of this test appears the same as that of your regular blood test results, the difference being that it shows your average blood glucose reading for up to the preceding three months. The test works by measuring your level of glycated (or glycosylated) haemoglobin, also known as Hb1c, HbA1c or haemoglobin A1c. Eye damage and kidney disease in diabetics has been found to be related to the glycation of haemoglobin.

Staying on top of HbA1c (or Average BG) in people with diabetes may well improve their treatment. Those who have persistent high blood sugar often show high levels of HbA1c. These high levels are often associated with long-term diabetes complications. Meanwhile, those with better glucose control will have a HbA1c within (or at least close to) the reference range of 4-6.5%.

This reading is only an average, though, and you should also be trying to avoid fluctuating blood sugars which move from very high to very low too often. Less damage is likely to be caused if you're able to keep your blood sugars relatively stable. We'll talk about these readings again later in the book.

Insulin Resistance Syndrome

In some cases, Type 2 diabetes is associated with insulin resistance syndrome. This condition is also known as metabolic syndrome, syndrome X, CHAOS (Australia), Reaven's syndrome or metabolic syndrome X.

What is Insulin Resistance Syndrome?

This condition exists in the form of a group of metabolic risk factors. The more dominant risk factors which characterise this syndrome seem to be insulin resistance and abdominal obesity. Other risk factors include premature ageing, hormonal imbalance and physical inactivity. It seems there could also be a genetic predisposition involved in the syndrome's development, meaning that if your parents had insulin resistance syndrome you have a higher chance of developing it yourself.

In these cases, the other risk factors like physical inactivity and excess body fat can increase the likelihood further. It's recommended by the National Heart, Lung and Blood Institute and the American Heart Association that this condition should be identified where an individual has at least three of the following:

1. Waist Circumference

    a. **Women:** Greater than or equal to 88cm (35 inches)

    b. **Men:** Greater than or equal to 102cm (40 inches)

2. Blood pressure: Greater than or equal to 130/85 mm Hg

3. Fasting glucose[1]: Greater than or equal to 10 mmols/L

4. Cholesterol levels (triglycerides): Greater than or equal to 150 mg/dL

    a. **Women:** Good (reduced HDL) cholesterol less than 50 mg/dL

    b. **Men:** Good (reduced HDL) cholesterol less than 40 mg/dL

---

1 *Fasting glucose is the name given to blood glucose tested at least 8 hours after you last ate, usually before breakfast.*

This condition appears to be complex, in that its cause is as yet unknown. It appears that the majority of patients with the syndrome are obese, have a high degree of insulin resistance, don't move around much and are older in age. It has not yet been fully determined whether insulin resistance and obesity are causes of the syndrome, or if they're simply symptoms of a condition which may affect the patient's cholesterol, blood sugar, blood pressure and weight.

Some research appears to show that some people have no way of knowing when they're full, and may overeat as a result. These people may become obese as their bodies simply don't register that they've eaten enough. However, even in these cases weight gain can be avoided through education and discipline, and encouragement to eat healthier foods, monitor the size of portions and avoid overeating.

Parents must be careful to implement these strategies early on, so that children learn to properly moderate their own eating habits in the future. In the meantime, we should watch out for the five key components of this condition, which are…

- High cholesterol
- High BMI (Body Mass Index)
- High hip to waist ratio
- High blood glucose
- High blood pressure

Other Forms of Diabetes

Brittle diabetes

Diabetes that is unusually difficult to control is often referred to as brittle diabetes. This condition is characterised by extreme, sudden drops in the blood sugar levels (hypos) which occur without warning and can render the individual unconscious. If you are concerned about having brittle diabetes, you or your doctor can request a screening process.

Maturity onset diabetes of the young (MODY)

This form of diabetes is rare, and occurs as a result of a flaw in a single gene. MODY exists in six different types - each caused by a different gene - and is diagnosed by genetic tests. Often, the condition is misdiagnosed as Type 1 diabetes when displayed by very young children generally under the age of one. Once these children receive the proper diagnosis, they are able to come off certain diabetes drugs (such as insulin) in favour of the correct treatment for their condition.

How will my diabetes affect others?

Of course, your diabetes diagnosis will affect you first and foremost, but it can also have a big impact on your friends, tutors, colleagues and family. It's generally argued that Type 1 diabetes is the more serious form of diabetes, with the possibility of a loss of consciousness or 'diabetic coma' if you fail to take the proper amount of insulin injections.

Friends

People are starting to be diagnosed with diabetes at an alarmingly high rate, with an estimated 2 million diabetics in the UK alone. You are far from being alone in your experiences. 25% of diabetics in the UK have Type 1 diabetes, which entails a large amounts of injections and blood tests which can make the condition pretty difficult to mask. While you may feel self-conscious about this initially, you will feel more comfortable with it as time goes on.

In the early days of the condition, some people find themselves most comfortable performing injections and blood tests in bathrooms rather than out in public. Similarly, those who are new to the condition may only wish to share this information with their closest and most trusted friends, and that's okay.

So long as your self-consciousness doesn't stop you from giving yourself the care and medication you need, there's nothing wrong with keeping this stuff on the down-low. However, this is not necessary: there's nothing wrong with standing where everyone can see you to do this.

It can be a good idea to make sure someone around you knows about your condition, just in case something goes wrong. Try to explain that you have diabetes, but that it isn't something to worry about provided you take the necessary medication. This means that if you do sense you're about to go hypo, it won't be completely unexpected if you need to ask for help (we'll talk more about hypo later in the book). There's also a chance that whoever you choose to tell will know other people with diabetes, and will know how to help in an emergency.

You'll be able to feel more comfortable and enjoy yourself more freely if you know that there's someone around you who understands your condition and knows what to do if you need help.

Family

Learning to live with any new medical condition can be a lonely experience, and can really take over your thoughts at the beginning. This means it's massively helpful to have your family on side as you begin to learn how to live with diabetes.

Eating the right food is a huge part of managing your diabetes. It may well be necessary to scrutinize the diet that you and your family enjoy. While a change in diet will only be essential to you, an improved diet will only serve to benefit your family as a whole.

Your Improved Diet: The Food Pyramid

The food pyramid is a guide that's used more in the United States than it is in the UK, but the information is relevant here all the same. The aim of this concept is to show how much food you are recommended to eat from each different group. As is shown in the diagram, you should try to eat a wide variety of different foods. A balanced diet is one which features foods from each group.

However, eating food from each category is not all there is to losing weight or eating more healthily. There are some foods of which you should eat a large amount (i.e. those at the wide base of the pyramid) and some you should eat only occasionally (those at the top). Try to eat foods of all different colours every day. Fruit and vegetables come in all different colours, and each has a different range of vital nutrients needed by your body.

Learning to live with any new medical condition can be a lonely experience, and can really take over your thoughts at the beginning. This means it's massively helpful to have your family on side as you begin to learn how to live with diabetes.

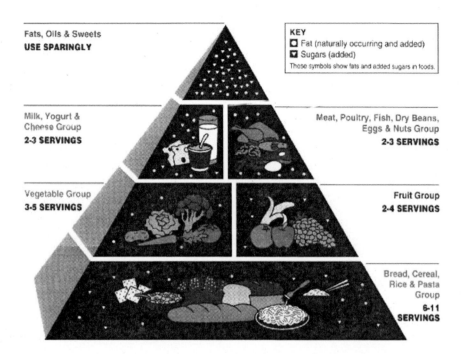

This is why dieticians may advise you to 'eat a rainbow'. If you're changing your diet not only to feel healthier but to lose weight also, you'll need to take into account the calories contained in each food item you consume. Try to search for fat-free or low-fat versions of your favourite foods, and to use fats like oil and butter as little as possible. Keep in mind that just because carbohydrates like pasta, cereals, rice and bread are at the bottom of the food pyramid, it doesn't mean you can eat an unlimited amount of these foods.

Don't forget that the food pyramid is just a guideline, and more detailed information can be given by your doctor or diabetes team. Have a certain amount of carbohydrates with each meal, but too many can lead to weight gain (and extra challenges for those with diabetes).

Work

If you have diabetes, you may also benefit from informing your colleagues so that you can rely on their understanding and help. This is especially important for certain specific jobs, which may have legal restrictions regarding this topic. If you're uncertain whether this applies to you, you can check Diabetes UK[2] who should be able to explain any legal requirements your employer may have, as well as your rights in different circumstances.

A lot of us really feel the need to keep our health to ourselves so as not to impose on those around us, but letting others know what's happening is a good idea in the long run. Even something as simple as a brief explanation of the condition and how it can affect your performance and daily life can be incredibly helpful. There's even a special section on job application forms where you can provide this information, and if you fill this in accurately it'll save you from having to bring up the topic yourself on other occasions.

If you have Type 1 diabetes, it's important that you keep a blood test machine to hand at all times in case you need to do a test at short notice. This is essential in the prevention and anticipation of hypos (hypoglycaemic episodes), when the level of sugar in your blood drops too low. These are also the main thing you'll want to warn colleagues about. Lots of people will have some understanding of what diabetes is, but won't necessarily know what to do if you have a hypo. It can be incredibly helpful to give them an idea of how they can help you if this happens.

In most cases, a person with diabetes will know how to manage their own hypos and this will be enough. But telling those around you can be a very useful backup if something goes wrong. We'll talk more about this later in the book. Don't be embarrassed about taking your medication, being careful with your food or doing blood tests in front of your colleagues. This something they'll get used to over time.

If your child has diabetes, it's important that you make sure your child's teachers are all fully informed. They will need to know what they should do to help your child, how they can tell if they're having a hypo, and what to do in that situation.

College and School

If your child has diabetes, it's important that you make sure your child's teachers are all fully informed. They will need to know what they should do to help your child, how they can tell if they're having a hypo, and what to do in that situation. While some children will have Type 2 diabetes, the vast majority have Type 1. It's likely that your child won't be the first in their school to have the condition, so many teachers will already be somewhat informed on the subject.

---

2 www.diabetes.org.uk

We'll discuss childhood diabetes in greater detail later in the book. Unsurprisingly, the most important thing to do for your diabetic child is to show them what they need to do to look after themselves properly. As a general rule, diabetes in children is more stable than that displayed in teenagers, as hormones can influence temperament and behaviour, how well medications can work as well as the blood sugar levels themselves.

Ensure your child is ready for college or school by keeping their equipment for diabetes management on hand at all times (including nighttime if necessary). They should always have access to their blood test machine and insulin kit or other medications. In most cases, a child's dosages can be administered before and after school, so they won't have to do any injections during the day.

It's likely that more injections will be needed as your child grows. This isn't a problem, and will only serve to give them more control over when and how they can eat and reflect the new needs of their changing bodies. Your child will most likely need to treat their diabetes for the rest of their lives, so it's important that they get used to living with it as soon as possible. It's possible they will feel worried their condition makes them different from their classmates, but it isn't necessarily a bad difference.

For the most part, this condition will just mean your child will need to be a bit more grown-up and responsible, at least when it comes to their health. By the time your child is going to college or university, they should have a good understanding of their diabetes. Some handy tips include…

- Letting new roommates or friends know about their condition;
- Keeping their insulin injection kit and blood test with them at all times;
- Being careful not to overextend themselves too often;
- Finding out what medical support is available in their new area and registering with a local doctor.

A number of organisations have useful information packs on what a school should know and what you need to do. These organisations include: Juvenile Diabetes Research Foundation (JDRF), the Insulin Dependent Diabetes Trust (IDDT), Diabetes Research and Wellness Foundation (DRWF) and Diabetes UK.

Children of different ages

A diabetes diagnosis will be tough no matter what age it happens, and there's no 'good' time for it to occur. It's likely that smaller children will have little or no idea of what's going on when it comes to diabetes. This issue is made all the more difficult by the fact that they may not be old enough to be able to explain how they're feeling, so you'll have to work it out based on their behaviour.

Older children, however, may have a stronger understanding of their medical condition and will have a better ability to process what they need to do to manage it. At this stage, provided your child has their diabetes kit with them, knows how to use it and can be trusted to do so, you can be fairly confident they'll be fine if you take a small step back. While diabetes was once a major source of self-consciousness, diabetes management equipment is now, faster, smaller and less obvious than it used to be so it's less likely to be a source of embarrassment.

Early blood test machines were around the size of a brick! By now, a lot of the diabetes equipment out there is actually pretty cool, and it's not unheard of for kids without diabetes to ask if they can try the blood test machine, just to see what it's like. This can be an interesting way for them to learn about the differences in everybody's bodies, as some kids will gush blood at a pinprick, while others will barely be able to squeeze out a drop.

It'll also give your kid's friends a chance to see what your child is dealing with, as they'll not only find out what taking a blood test is like, but will also see the difference between their own readings and those of your child. Rest assured that this is completely safe for them to do, provided nobody shares a lancet. One of the main things you'll need to look out for in your child with diabetes is irritability, but this can be difficult in age groups (like toddlers and teenagers) where irritability is not uncommon.

Following the diagnosis, the easiest way to know for sure what level their blood sugar is at is by testing it. Your child won't be happy with it, but it's important that you know if you should be scolding them for being naughty or giving them a chocolate biscuit for their blood sugar! Many professionals believe that teenagers have tendencies either toward being very good or very bad at diabetes management, with very few falling in between.

This is generally because kids this age are very prone to being self-conscious. Many teens feel it'll be difficult to fit in if they're constantly taking injections and blood tests, and being 'difficult' or 'weird' about what and when they eat.

What have we learned?

Diabetes will have an impact on your life, but it doesn't have to be too extreme. Making sure those around you have an understanding of your condition will make things a lot easier for everyone in both the long and short terms. In time, it'll become something you won't need to think twice about. It'll all become second nature. Pay attention to the different ways in which your body might react to different types of food and drink.

Taking plenty of exercise is a good change for anyone to make, not just people who want to lose a bit of weight. Try to incorporate it into each day as much as you can, even if this just means taking the stairs instead of the elevator. Get into the habit of frequent blood testing. It's not a difficult thing to do, but putting it off can have drastic consequences. Try to gather as much information as you can about the type of diabetes you have, and work through it slowly and carefully.

This can be a lot of reading, so take the time to digest it slowly.

2

Blood Tests

A Brief History

The impact of intensive therapy on long-term diabetes complications was assessed through a 10-year study. This research was carried out by the National Institute of Diabetes and Digestive and Kidney Diseases in America between 1983 and 1993. It was known as the Diabetes Control and Complications Trial (DCCT), and clearly illustrated that the close control of insulin-dependent diabetes delayed or prevented the development of long-term diabetes complications.

Blood tests (and in the case of Type 1 diabetes frequent doses of insulin) are part of this intensive management, and are essential if you want to avoid complications such as kidney, nerve and eye damage.

Blood Test Basics

Blood Glucose Meters (or blood test machines)

Thanks to the massive range of personal blood glucose meters that you can choose from today, you're sure to find one to suit your needs (we'll talk about diabetes equipment in greater detail later in the book). These tools are invaluable when it comes to helping control your condition.

They can generally be bought in a pharmacy for less than £20, which is a very low price when compared to your life, health and peace of mind.

Whichever you choose, you'll easily get the hang of it very quickly as they're very simple to use. You may even be given a free blood glucose meter by your diabetes nurse following diagnosis, and will be able to get plenty of advice from the same person. Your device will come with instructions, and may well have information about helplines you can call if you're struggling.

A lot of modern designs have built-in memories, so you can access your results later or transfer them to a PC if you don't have time to record them straight away. For those with Type 1 diabetes, it can be a good idea to get a spare blood glucose meter if possible. It's useful to have one with you wherever you are during the day - be that in your work cubicle, glove compartment or bag - as well as at home.

It's also comforting to know you have a backup and won't be stuck if something happens to your other meter.

Lancets

Blood tests can be a pain, but they aren't the end of the world. Lancets are devices used for sampling blood, and work by pricking the skin to obtain samples. Over the years, this technology has improved to an impressive degree, with lancets which are much sharper (and therefore less painful) and adjustable in depth. This means you can test the blood of a thick-skinned workman or a young child and it'll work just as well.

In most cases, you'll just end up using whichever lancing device comes with your blood glucose meter. That said, some people choose to keep their original lancing device even when they get a new meter, specifically buy meters that come with their preferred lancing devices or simply buy a lancing device on its own. All of these options are fine, and it's important that you just do what works best for you.

Blood testing sites

Many people choose the ends of their fingers as the main sites for blood testing, even though these sites are known to be very sensitive. It's generally a good idea to use the edges of your fingertips rather than the very tips of your fingers, as these are usually slightly less sensitive. Some devices work fine with ATS or alternative testing sites. These include the forearm and other easily accessed areas.

In small children, earlobes may be used as blood testing sites. Whichever you go for, it's not a good idea to use the exact same site over and over again. As with your sites for insulin injection, it's best to change things up every now and then to stop yourself from getting very sore. Even just changing the finger you use each time can prevent this.

Accessing Blood Test Strips

Anyone with Type 1 diabetes should be able to get their blood test sensors on a prescription. This may also be an option if you have Type 2 diabetes, but you'll have to discuss it with your GP. Some GPs only distribute a limited amount of blood test sensors through prescription. If you're struggling to get sensors this way, you can contact Diabetes UK for guidance.

Blood test frequency

For those with Type 1 (insulin-dependent) diabetes, it's generally a good idea to try and test your blood sugar a minimum of three times per day, usually before every meal. Eating less than you usually would, being ill, travelling, exercising more than normal or any other changes to your routine are also good reasons to check your blood glucose levels.

These amounts are reduced for those with Type 2 diabetes, who may only have to test their blood sugar once each day as they can use oral medication alongside their insulin (or instead of insulin) to manage their diabetes. If you don't need medication and can manage your blood sugar through diet and exercise, you may only need to test your blood sugar once every week.

Blood Tests During Pregnancy

When you're pregnant, it becomes extra-important to test your blood frequently, and many doctors will encourage you to be even stricter with your targets than usual. If you want to keep the risk to your developing baby as low as possible, it's best to keep your blood sugar levels as close to normal as you possibly can, even prior to your child's conception. If you're good at adjusting your insulin doses in response to frequent blood sugar tests then try to do this to help you meet your new targets.

As often as possible, you'll want the morning blood test you take before breakfast (fasting blood glucose) to be around 6.0 mmols/L. For the rest of the day, it's best to aim for blood sugars below

8.0 mmols/L. Always keep in mind that pregnancy will alter your daily energy requirements. The ways in which your body processes your insulin doses and the food you eat may well mean that you need to change your set patterns for the duration of your pregnancy.

It's not all bad news, though, as in many cases people actually find control easier to reach and maintain during pregnancy.

Blood test results

Normal blood sugar levels for people who don't have diabetes fall somewhere between 4.0 and 8.0 mmols/L (millimoles per litre). However, for those who do have diabetes these 'normal' results may not occur quite so often. If your blood sugar falls under 4.0 mmols/L this means you have low blood sugar and are hypoglycaemic. Meanwhile, if your level is higher than 8.0 mmols/L then you have high blood sugar and are hyperglycaemic.

Gaining good control over your blood sugar levels is the most effective way of avoiding damage to your eyes, feet and kidneys, or any other unpleasant complications that are associated with diabetes. Your diabetes team should recommend a certain amount of blood tests, and you should stay as close to that as you possibly can, and write down all of your results so that you can identify any patterns.

Try not to be overly worried or discouraged by bad results, as everyone gets these from time to time. One of the main downsides of all these blood tests is that you're getting new information and updates constantly, and it can be difficult to make out what is worth noting when you get overloaded by so many readings. You need to get used to reading your results with your doctor's cap on: if your results aren't 'normal', then why? Why is your blood sugar high? Why is it low?

Gaining good control over your blood sugar levels is the most effective way of avoiding damage to your eyes, feet and kidneys, or any other unpleasant complications that are associated with diabetes.

You can't hope to properly improve your results until you fully understand them. Also keep in mind that more tests doesn't necessarily mean better health: taking three or four tests each day should be fine, not one every half hour. Try to spot all the patterns you can. For example, if you find your blood sugar is often high after breakfast time, you may need more insulin with this meal.

Writing down every reading can be very helpful for this, especially if you remember to take down times and events with each reading.

Hypoglycaemia (hypos)

Hypos are more or less inevitable for those with diabetes, no matter how good you are at controlling your condition. In fact, they seem to be extra-common in those who are well controlled. However, if you're well controlled this also likely means you'll have an understanding of hypo symptoms and a good idea of what strategies work to deal with it properly.

If you have your diabetes under control, it means your blood test results mostly fall within the recommended 4.0-8.0 mmols/L range. This can be a pretty small target to try and aim for, especially if you have Type 1 diabetes and need to control it through blood tests and insulin injections. It's easy to find yourself falling close to or slightly under the lower guideline of 4.0 mmols/L.

Interpreting your results

It's easiest to interpret your results if you write them all down in the same space. This doesn't simply mean writing down the results of each blood test, but also any medication you're on, what dosages you're taking, the time of day, what you've been doing and how well you've been eating. You may then wish to discuss these results with your diabetes team, but it's also important that you gain your own understanding of your condition.

You need to really know what's happening with your blood sugar levels, especially if you're going through a particularly difficult time or have only recently been diagnosed with diabetes. It may seem like a sharp learning curve, but don't worry too much. Here are some factors you should consider when trying to work out your blood readings, especially if they come out high or low.

- **What time is it?** Your blood test records are likely to be lower before mealtimes, or higher if you've recently eaten.

- **What medication have you taken?** If you get a string of high or low readings, it may suggest you need to take more medication. For example, if you're always high before lunchtime it may mean you need more medication with breakfast.

- **What have you eaten lately?** Your results will reflect the nature of what you last ate, and how recently it was. We'll discuss this in greater detail later.

Change to HbA1c Reporting

HbA1c tests are used to measure someone's average blood glucose levels over the previous 2-3 months to find out how well their long-term diabetes control has been working. It's recommendedthat those with diabetes receive a HbA1c test at least once each year. The way in which HbA1c levels are measured in those with diabetes changed in October 2011. At this point, it was decided by the Department of Health that HbA1c levels should be measured in millimoles per mole (mmol/mol) rather than percentage unites.

Adopting a global approach in the way HbA1c levels are measured will be of great benefit as it will now become easier for international laboratories and research trials to compare results across the world.

However, we must ensure that this change does not impact on people with diabetes. It is vital that both clinicians and patients understand the new measurements to ensure the way they manage their condition and the care they receive is not compromised. There is still time to familiarise yourself with the new measurements before the change takes place and Diabetes UK has produced an online HbA1c converter tool to help people adjust to the new measurements[3].

More information as well as a handy conversion tool can be found through Diabetes UK[4]. The conversion tool produced by Diabetes UK was designed to help healthcare professionals and people with diabetes to familiarise themselves with these changed measurements, and to make sure those with diabetes would not experience issues with their treatment while these systems were changed.

As explained by the charity, 'Diabetes UK welcomes the change in reporting but is concerned people may still be unfamiliar with the new measurements.'

---

3 *Quote from Natasha Marshland, Clinical Advisor to Diabetes UK.*
4 *www.diabetes.org.uk/HbA1c*

What have we learned?

Make a point of talking to your diabetes nurse or GP about which blood test machine they'd recommend and how often you should be testing yourself. You need to take proper care of yourself at all times and schedule your blood tests carefully, because your diabetes isn't going to change its schedule just because you're busy. For those with Type 1 diabetes (and those with Type 2 who take insulin), it's generally a good idea to test before eating.

Try not to feel too guilty if you get disappointing results in a blood test. Everyone gets this from time to time. All you can do is learn how to figure out why your blood sugar is high or low, and how to avoid this in the future. It can be a good idea to keep a blood test diary, especially if you're struggling with your diabetes control or have only recently been diagnosed.

3

Which Medications can Help?

Diabetes Management

The most important thing you can keep in mind here is that diabetes management is not a sprint, it's a marathon. Those with Type 2 diabetes generally display two main problems: The cells in their bodies don't take in as much glucose as they should, and they aren't able to make enough insulin for themselves. Fortunately, there are drugs available which can help to manage Type 2 diabetes and allow diabetics to maintain control over their blood glucose.

In some cases, doctors recommend that you take more than one of these types of drugs. It's also possible that after taking them for a number of years, their effectiveness may be reduced in which case you may need to change your prescription. Please keep in mind that the information we provide here is only a guide, and you must talk to your doctor before taking any type of medication.

Sulfonylureas

Of the medications available, these are the oldest tablets. Drugs such as tolazamide (Tolinase) have been around since the 1950s and are still available on prescription. This class also includes newer drugs such as glipizide extended release (Glucotrol XL), glyburide (Diabeta, Micronase), glimepiride (Amaryl) and glipizide (Glucotrol). These medications lower the glucose level by allowing the pancreas to release more insulin, but are often associated with hypoglycaemia. A lot of these medications only stay effective for a couple of years.

Starch Blockers

Two of the most commonly prescribed starch blockers (also known as alpha-glucosidase inhibitors) are acarbose (Precose) and miglitol (Glyset). These are drugs which block the breakdown of starches (such as those found in potatoes, pasta and bread) in the intestine in order to lower the body's blood glucose levels. They also inhibit the breakdown of certain sugars, such as regular granulated sugar.

In order to effectively slow digestion and inhibit the rise of glucose in the blood, these drugs need to be taken at the start of each meal. The can be prescribed in conjunction with other diabetes medications, though they can cause gas and diarrhoea.

Meglitinides

These include nateglinide (Starlix) and repaglinide (Prandin). As with starch blockers, these drugs should be taken before each meal. They work by causing the pancreas to produce higher amounts of insulin relative to the amount of glucose in the blood. For increased effectiveness, meglitinides may be used in combination with some other oral medications.

Insulin

In the United States, manufacturers advertise their insulin and devices on television, making it the patient's decision to discuss and incorporate it into their diabetes treatment. In the UK, this link does not exist, so it falls on the doctor and patient to find all the information necessary. For those with Type 1 diabetes, insulin injections are an unavoidable fact of life if you wish to control your condition.

However, those with Type 2 diabetes are also being put on insulin therapy with increasing frequency in order to treat their diabetes. Insulin therapy can come with a large amount of medical equipment - lancing devices, insulin pens, insulin pumps, needles and blood test machines - but by now these are all of great quality. Needles and lancing devices especially have become sharper, smaller and less painful, so you couldn't have chosen a better time to be diagnosed!

It can take time to get used to insulin therapy, but it is a reliable way of controlling your condition so the pros far outweigh the cons. Try to keep in mind that ending up on insulin is not a sign of failure, or that your diabetes is getting worse. It's simply a sign that insulin therapy is the treatment which will work best for you at this time. Your blood test results will act as proof that your new treatment is helping, and is well worth all of this extra work.

Short-acting and long-acting insulin

Different types of insulin have been made to treat those with diabetes. Each type has its own pattern of release, and works slightly differently from the other types. Short-acting insulin is the name given to insulins that begin working quickly, do their job and then become inactive within just a few hours. These includes insulins like Novo Nordisk's Novo Rapid and Eli Lilly's Humalog.

As a general rule, short-acting insulins will begin to work within 10-20 minutes of injection and will start wearing off after around two hours. This system is designed to mimic the release pattern that occurs naturally in non-diabetic bodies around meal times. Injections of short-acting insulin are generally taken alongside a meal. But the body doesn't only need insulin at mealtimes - it needs it at all times.

This is why people with diabetes are likely to take a long-acting type of insulin as well, to work alongside the short-acting mealtime insulin. Long-acting insulins include Novo Nordisk's Levemir and Sanofi-Aventis's Lantus. By taking this

It can take time to get used to insulin therapy, but it is a reliable way of controlling your condition so the pros far outweigh the cons. Try to keep in mind that ending up on insulin is not a sign of failure, or that your diabetes is getting worse.

'peakless' insulin (sometimes referred to as 24-hour insulin), the diabetic has insulin present throughout the day. Often, if a person with Type 2 diabetes finds they need to take insulin, it will be a long-acting type.

Beginning to take insulin may mean that drugs you previously used are no longer doing their jobs, but it doesn't mean your condition is getting worse. Insulin therapy is only suggested if it seems to be the best way to avoid potential diabetes complications by achieving better blood sugar control.

DPP-4 inhibitors

These include:

- Saxagliptin
- Alogliptin + Metformin
- Linagliptin + Metformin
- Saxagliptin + Metformin
- Linagliptin
- Alogliptin

These are a newer class of drugs which work by blocking the action of DPP-4, an enzyme which breaks down the hormone incretin. These hormones are instrumental in helping the body to produce additional insulin only when it is needed and prevent the liver from producing glucose when it is not needed. Incretins are released throughout the day, with increased levels at meal times.

Thiazolidinediones

Pioglitazone is the only remaining tablet in this group. This drug is taken once or twice each day either with or without food. It allows the insulin produced by the body to work more effectively by improving insulin sensitivity and reducing insulin resistance. It also works to protect the cells in the pancreas in order to allow them to produce insulin for longer. Pioglitazone can be used in combination with a metformin or sulphonylurea, in combination with both or on its own.

If the individual is intolerant to metformin, this drug can also be used in combination with insulin.

Biguanides

These medications work by altering the production of glucose through digestion. Unlike sulfonylureas, they do not cause hypoglycaemia but can help with weight loss and lowering cholesterol. Some drugs may cause diarrhoea, but this can be improved by taking the doses with food. This is the type of drug most commonly prescribed for Type 2 diabetes. Two of the more well known of these drugs are metformin extended release (Glucophage XR) and metformin (Glucophage).

Metformin is generally taken twice each day, and primarily works to lower blood glucose levels by reducing the amount of glucose the liver produces. The drug also makes muscle tissue more sensitive to insulin, lowering blood glucose levels by increasing the amount of glucose absorbed.

GLP-1s

The hormone GLP-1 (glucagon-like peptide-1) is generally secreted within the intestine. It's known to delay and protract carbohydrate absorption by inhibiting gastric secretion and motility (so thatyou stay fuller for longer), and also seems to restore pancreatic beta cells' glucose sensitivity. For those with Type 2 diabetes, injectables are now available including liraglutide (Victoza) and exenatide (Byetta), which are usually applied with an injection once each day.

Using these injections does not necessarily mean you'll need to do daily blood tests.

Other Drugs

Angiotensin-Converting Enzyme Inhibitors

Angiotensin-converting enzyme inhibitors (more commonly known as ACE Inhibitors) are a drug group usually used when treating congestive heart failure and high blood pressure (hypertension). You may be prescribed this medication to prevent the development of kidney disease or if you begin to show protein in your urine (signs of renal disease).

Statins

Like ACE inhibitors, statins are an important class of drugs as they have been found to reduce the likelihood of death by stroke or heart attack. These are tablets designed to lower your cholesterol. They work by blocking the enzyme in the liver which is responsible for producing cholesterol, causing less to be made, and lowering the level that reaches your bloodstream. Your doctor will consider giving these to you if you have diabetes and are at risk of suffering a stroke or heart attack.

Diet and Pill Therapy

Following your diabetes diagnosis, you're going to need to properly examine your snacking habits and diet. 'Diet' is simply the word for all the things you drink and eat, and is not the same thing as 'being on a diet'. As Type 1 diabetes is a genetic condition, it can affect even those who have a perfectly healthy diet and lifestyle. However, the vast majority of Type 2 diabetes cases (around 80%) are tied to being overweight, so with this condition you may well be introduced to dieth therapy straight away (often along with some pills to help control certain symptoms).

If diet therapy doesn't deliver the desired results, insulin therapy may be introduced to help with blood glucose control. Type 2 diabetes can also be treated by other, non-insulin injectable medicines, as we have discussed above. 'Success' is determined based on blood test results, and going on insulin doesn't mean you have 'failed' at controlling your condition. This is simply another tool you have to try and control your health.

Insulin therapy

Insulin comes in a number of different forms and brands, but your diabetes team will be able to offer guidance on which you should be using. Ask as many questions as you feel is necessaryabout your dosage and medication, but be careful and patient. It can take time for your medication and you to 'settle down'. Finding the right dosages can take a while. Your dosage may also change according to your time of life, age and other factors over the years.

The main types of insulin available include…

- **Rapid-acting insulin:** This lasts for a few hours and begins working within 15 minutes.

- **Intermediate-acting insulin:** This begins working within 2-4 hours, as it is mixed with a substance which causes the body to absorb the insulin more slowly.

- **Basal (long-acting) insulin:** This is often referred to as 24-hour insulin, as its influence and release tend to last a full day. It acts in a way that is pretty much stable all day.

- **Short-acting insulin:** This lasts for a few hours and begins working within 30-45 minutes.

Most adults who take insulin go for a short-acting and a long-acting insulin. This is because this is the best way to imitate the functioning of a non-diabetic body. People who don't have diabetes will have a certain amount of insulin in their body at all times, but will have a larger amount present when they eat. Sugar levels are measured constantly by the brain's pituitary gland.

If blood sugar levels are too low, the body raises them by producing glucagon. If they're too high, it lowers them by releasing insulin. If you're using insulin, you're doing the work of the pituitary gland manually by using a blood test machine. You can then work out how much insulin you need and administer that amount.

Which insulin is best for me?

This is something your diabetes team will work out when talking to you, but they'll usually be taking the following factors into account:

- Any other health requirements you have, such as diet, other medications and activity levels.

- How old you are.

- How you have responded to insulin in the past.

- The insulin's action and how this will suit you, including its peak in terms of action, how long it lasts and how quickly it will begin to work.

- Your willingness to take multiple injections, and your ability to perform glucose monitoring (NB. If you have Type 1 diabetes, you have no choice here. You will have to inject insulin and take frequent blood tests).

How to store your insulin

It's vital you know how to look after your insulin, both by using it properly and storing it correctly. This medication has a use-by-date, and you need to check this carefully before starting a new cartridge or bottle of insulin. As a general rule,

It's vital you know how to look after your insulin, both by using it properly and storing it correctly.

when it's not in use your insulin should be stored in the fridge. When it is in use (either in your bag or in an insulin pen) you should try to keep it out of sunlight and store it in a dry place at room temperature.

Talk to your diabetes nurse or GP for advice on storing your insulin, and always read the instructions that come with the container. Insulin should never be frozen as this will deactivate it and make it useless. High temperatures can also impair its functionality. Once your insulin has been opened, it's a good idea to use it within 28 days, whether or not it has been refrigerated. We'll talk more about keeping insulin cool later in the book.

How should I take my insulin?

Many doctors will recommend taking insulin around 20 minutes before eating your meal. This will work in most cases, but if you're eating out somewhere new it may be a better idea to wait and see your food before deciding on your dosage. This delay will be fine, as digestion doesn't begin straight away so your insulin will generally still have started working by the time your food has started releasing its energy.

The time at which you take your insulin - be that straight before beginning your meal or 20 minutes in advance - should also vary depending on the type of insulin you take as some start working straight away and others take a little time. Check out our guide to different types a few pages back. Once you've taken your insulin, it's in your body and will do exactly what it's designed to do whether you want it to or not.

You don't want to order your food and take your insulin, only to discover that the meal you're about to eat has a different amount of carbs to what you expected. While this can be an absolute pain when it happens, it's not the end of the world. In most cases you'll be able to order some extra bread to use up your extra insulin, or not finish your meal if you find you haven't taken enough.

For more advice on taking your insulin, talk to your diabetes nurse or GP.

Human or animal insulin

Most of the insulin available today is manufactured by pharmaceutical companies and is referred to as 'human insulin'. In the past however, the only insulin available was animal insulin which was extracted from the pancreases of cows and pigs. While these *bovine* and *porcine* insulins are very rarely given out, they are still available. Certain insulin users claimed they experienced serious side effects on moving from animal to human insulin, though this is more than likely as a result of incorrect dosage calculations when trying to convert one type to the other.

Because you need to take less human insulin than you would animal insulin, failure to convert your dosage properly could easily cause horrible, huge hypos which would make anyone uneasy about the change. That said, today most people are able to take human insulin very successfully.

Damaged insulin

If your short-acting insulin appears lumpy, crystallised or cloudy, it may be inactive and you should not take it without first seeking proper medical advice. Long-acting insulins are generally cloudy in appearance, but you should still look out for crystals or clumping as signs of damage. If you are concerned, talk to your doctor.

Insulin dosage

This will be a vital part of your control over your blood sugar levels and general diabetes management. If you do it right, your blood test results should fall in the recommended 'normal' range of between 4.0-8.0 mmols/L, or a little higher if you've just eaten. It's important that you keep trying even if your readings fall outside of this range and don't get disheartened, as getting it right can be very difficult and will take some practice.

If you're able to master blood sugar control, you'll reduce your likelihood of experiencing diabetes complications, which will become a big part of your everyday life. One of the major tools people with diabetes use to do this is 'carbohydrate counting'. The idea is to keep track of the amount of carbohydrates you're about to consume, and to plan your insulin dose accordingly.

The dose you take will also depend on the following factors:

- The result of your blood test.
- If you plan on doing exercise soon.
- What food you're about to eat, and how much.

There are many guides available describing how much insulin you should take with carbohydrates, but a simple rule is to take one unit of insulin for every 10g of carbohydrate. This is something we'll discuss in greater detail later in the book, but do remember that your dose is affected by variables other than carbohydrates, including your height and weight. Everyone with diabetes needs to take a different amount of insulin, and you may find that you really need to take four units of insulin for every 10g of carbohydrate.

If your short-acting insulin appears lumpy, crystallised or cloudy, it may be inactive and you should not take it without first seeking proper medical advice.

Learning about your reactions to different foods will help you get used to which foods you'll need to avoid and which will mean you need to adjust your insulin dosage. If the carbohydrate you're about to eat is combined with fat, as with chips, the fat will also alter the ways in which the food is absorbed. You may find that you'll need a higher dosage of insulin for meals like this, or that you'll need to take an extra injection a little later on.

In the UK, there are education programmes for people with diabetes which feature information on counting carbohydrates. These are called DESMOND (for those with Type 2 diabetes) and DAFNE (for those with Type 1). We'll talk about these in greater detail later on, but you could alsotalk to your diabetes team to find out how you can access them and whether they would be helpful for you.

Insulin: A Factfile

- While researchers are currently working to create functioning insulin pills, this medication cannot currently be swallowed as it is destroyed by stomach acid.

- The body will absorb insulin at different rates depending on where you inject it. The best site is generally the belly as insulin is absorbed the most consistently here.

- Don't inject into the same part of your body all the time, it's best to rotate your sites as much as possible. If you use the same site each time it will get painful, as you're damaging your body with repeated injections. This can also affect the rate at which your insulin is absorbed.

- If you combine insulins for an injection, you should inject this within 5 minutes of mixing them.

- Good injection sites include the inner and outer thighs, the stomach, the top of the buttocks and the upper arm.

- Do not inject your short-acting insulins in the same site as your long-acting, as this may negatively affect the absorption capabilities of both. Consider using your arms or belly for short-acting doses and your thighs for long-acting insulin.

- Current delivery methods for insulin include insulin pens, insulin pumps, jet injectors and needle-and-syringe injections. Attempts have been made to create an inhaled insulin option, resulting in the creation of Exubera. This delivered insulin into the nose by a pump, but did not gain popularity as the pump was very large and drew a lot of unwanted attention to users.

What have we learned?

It takes a bit of time to get used to any new medication, and those prescribed to diabetics are no different. Whatever medication you're given, give yourself a bit of time and space to figure out the right dosage for you. Follow the instructions on your medications regarding storage, and make sure they're safely out of the reach of children. In the case of insulin, you'll need to avoid extreme temperatures (hot or cold).

When travelling, bring insulin in your carry-on luggage is it may freeze if left in the hold. If you need any advice about medication, talk to your GP. Don't stop taking your insulin, even if you're unwell or off your food for any other reason. You can reduce your dosage if needs be, just don't stop taking it altogether.

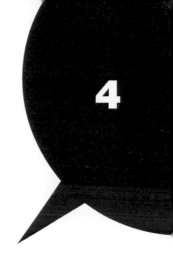

4

Treating Hypers and Hypos

ypoglycaemia (very low blood sugar levels) or hyperglycaemia (very high blood sugar levels) can easily occur in those with diabetes and will need treatment urgently. It can be easy to get the two words confused, but if in doubt remember that 'low' goes with 'hypo'. Diabetics with low blood sugar may be said to be 'going hypo' or 'having a hypo'. Blood tests can be used to find out if you're having a hyper or hypo.

Keep in mind that not all blood tests with results over 8.0 mmols/L will need urgent action. If your result is just a bit higher than normal, it's best to wait a while before taking any extra insulin, in case the level lowers by itself. In order to treat a hyper (over 8.0 mmols/L) you'll likely need to take pills or insulin, while for hypoglycaemia (under 4.0 mmols/L) you may administer some form of sugar.

People with diabetes will describe hypoglycaemia in a few different ways, with many explaining it as 'feeling a bit wobbly'. It's common for someone to behave strangely while having a hypo, as the condition is often linked with difficulty seeing, sudden irritability and giddiness.

Ketoacidosis and Hyperglycaemia

When your blood sugar levels become too high, this is called hyperglycaemia. The symptoms of a hyper are generally less dramatic than hypos, unless you fail to treat them in which case you may end up in hospital. Common symptoms for this include drowsiness, needing to urinate a lot, and generally feeling thirsty and unwell. Always remember that not every blood test with results of 8.0 mmols/L or higher needs to be treated straight away.

Even if your result reaches 9.0-10 mmols/L, it's best to give it time to drop by itself before taking extra insulin. If action is required, it'll vary depending on the medications you take. Many cases simply call for a small shot of insulin. It's common for people with diabetes to find confusing or unexpected high blood sugars pretty upsetting, especially if they've been working hard to control their blood sugar levels.

An unaddressed hyper can result in a diabetic coma (or sugar coma) as a result of ketoacidosis, a process that occurs in the body when blood sugars reach very high levels. This involves releasing energy for the body to use by breaking down body fat. Put simply, this is your body initiating an emergency back-up plan which is not designed to work for very long, and will become toxic to the body in time.

Without treatment you may lose consciousness and will need to be hospitalised to regain consciousness and control of your blood sugar. Ketoacidosis can also release ketones as a

by-product, which may affect brain function if allowed to build up. Some guidelines suggest that if blood test results come back as more than 12 mmols/L, the diabetic should also test for ketones.

There are test machines out there designed specifically to test for ketones. There are even blood test machines which can test for ketones as well as blood sugar levels, using different strips for each. These include the Abbott Xceed and the

Menarini LX Plus. It's ironic that although this condition is caused by high blood sugar levels, its symptoms occur because the body is unable to access all of this sugar. For that, it needs insulin.

Without medical intervention, a patient with this condition can easily just waste away and become dehydrated. This is what many people with diabetes would die of before the discovery of insulin in 1921. At the end of the day, though, if you have fairly good control over your diabetes ketones will not be something you need to worry about. It can also be helpful to remember that if you're unwell it's common to have slightly higher blood sugars than usual.

This doesn't mean you should stop taking your medication. If you are eating less than usual you may need to reduce your insulin dosage for the time being, but it's vital that you don't stop taking it entirely. Your body needs insulin to survive. If you start getting ketone readings unexpectedly, this is something you can talk over with your diabetes team. The only way to treat ketoacidosis is by regaining control of your diabetes and keeping your sugar between 4.0 and 10 mmols/L.

Your best plan of action is to let those around you know what will happen in the event your blood sugar levels drop, and what should be done.

Handling a Hypo

Hypoglycaemia is right at the other end of the scale and is when you have a low blood sugar. One of the main things you'll need to get used to is properly handling a hypo without overdoing the treatment. One thing that can make this incredibly difficult is that a hypo can make you feel incredibly disoriented and blur your understanding of what needs to be done. You may find it difficult to make the best decision for your health, to explain what you need or even to understand what is happening to you.

Some hypos can be more difficult to manage than others, with a reading of 3.0 mmols/L or even less occurring very suddenly. Your best plan of action is to let those around you know what will happen in the event your blood sugar levels drop, and what should be done. Many people with diabetes will reach a stage where they know exactly what they need to do to fix their blood sugar level.

Even in this case, you should try to keep everyone in the loop so that they can be helpful in this scenario rather than simply getting in the way. For example, maybe for them a reading of 2.5 mmols/L can be brought to healthy levels with a glass of juice and some chocolate, while higher readings will only require the juice. If the people you're with also know this, they'll understand what's happening if you suddenly ask for a cup of juice and try to help rather than asking unnecessary questions.

Hypos: Vocabulary and Definition

Healthy blood sugar levels will fall between 4.0-8.0 mmols/L. This means a hypo occurs when your blood sugar falls under the minimum recommended 4.0 mmols/L, and your best bet is to make sure this is the lowest reading you'll get. In fact, some people with diabetes aim to 'make 5 the floor' and make 5.0 mmols/L the lowest reading they get, eating a biscuit or something sugary any time they reach this level.

A big part of living with diabetes is simply trying to keep your head above water. It's not easy to deal with this condition, and your best bet is to do everything in your power to keep hypos and hypers to a minimum. Mild hypos might have readings of around 3.6 mmols/L, while severe hypos can be so low that your blood test meter won't be able to give you a proper reading. In this case, the meter will most likely just say 'low'.

In some cases, a hypo will come with 'good' symptoms which will make it clear what is happening. However, hypos should really be avoided as much as possible as they are unpleasant experiences which can affect blood test results for a few hours. If you ask anyone with diabetes, they'll be able to describe what it feels like to have a hypo - highly-strung, battling a strong urge to eat anything you can get your hands on, struggling to concentrate, feeling shaky.

What you experience when your blood sugar is low, and how you deal with that situation, will vary from person to person. Some other factors that may play a part might include where you are, how active you've been recently, what you can get your hands on quickly, what you've eaten lately and what seems to have caused your hypo.

The lower your reading, the more sugar you need to raise your blood sugar. Liquids will work faster to pull you out of your hypo than solids, so your best bet for a first step is something like orange juice, a smoothie or a GlucoGel product.

Treating a Hypo

The rule here is fairly simple: The lower your reading, the more sugar you need to raise your blood sugar. Liquids will work faster to pull you out of your hypo than solids, so your best bet for a first step is something like orange juice, a smoothie or a GlucoGel product. Before sugars can be released from solid foods, they need to be digested to a certain extent. This means they will do the job, but will just take a little longer than liquid alternatives.

Treatment for a hypo is often referred to as a 'sugar source' because anything sugary can be used, although some are more effective than others. Similarly, crunchable or chewable sweets will deliver sugar far more quickly than boiled sweets, as they can be broken down more quickly. No product can officially claim the title of 'hypo treatment' unless it's been clinically tested for this purpose, something which has happened with very few products indeed.

Substances like soft drinks, chocolate, orange juice and sugar have not been clinically tested, but any person with diabetes will be able to tell you that they do the job when you need to come out of a hypo.

Hypos: Ten Tips to Remember

- Keep stashes of sugar sources everywhere - in your car door, in your briefcase, rucksack or handbag, in a desk drawer at work and next to your bed. Make it clear to those around you that these aren't to be used by anyone but you, as they will be needed in an emergency.

- If you feel like a hypo is on the horizon, try to do a blood test if at all possible. For many people, feelings of anxiety can easily be confused with warning signs for a hypo. The important difference is that while sugar will help a hypo, it'll be no help if what you're feeling is anxiety unrelated to your condition. Make sure you know what you're dealing with here.

- Whatever you use to treat your hypo, read the label carefully. You need to know how much energy you are putting into your body.

- Try to keep a record of all of your hypos so that you can spot any patterns that emerge. If you find that you seem to get hypos around the same time every day or two, it might suggest that you need to alter your medication or change your meal habits and diet.

- Keep sugar nearby so that you can deal with any hypo as quickly as possible. This will also save you from having to go to another room or up or down stairs while hypo.

Preparation is everything. Remember to replace any sugar sources you use, as you don't want to realise you've run out when you've already started your next hypo!

- Keep a second blood test machine in your bedroom. This will come in handy if you wake up feeling hypo, or are struggling to fall asleep and are worried it's because of low blood sugars. Ask for a spare at a clinic or buy one yourself - you should be able to find one for less than £20 at any pharmacy.

- After treating your hypo, give yourself 10 minutes before taking another blood test. This will show you if you need to treat your hypo further.

- Do a third test after about an hour. At this point, you may find that you've pushed yourself too far the other way and need some insulin to bring your blood sugar back down. Be careful with this, though! Too much insulin too soon may just cause another hypo.

- Try to treat your hypo with a combination of fast-acting sugary foods (like fruit juice, soft drinks and sweets) and more long-term solutions like bread or biscuits which will release sugars over a longer period. Don't overdo it, though!

- Explain signs and symptoms to your close friends and family members, and say how they can help you if you're having a hypo. Make sure at least one of your work colleagues knows what to do in the event of a hypo.

Hypos and Pregnancy

While this is advice diabetics should follow already, it's especially important that your partner, coworkers and family members know how to give you a shot of glucagon in the unlikely event that you very suddenly have very low blood sugar. Make sure you're always wearing some identification that will tell people you have diabetes, such as a MediPAL or Medic Alert. If youhave diabetes, your best plan is to try to be very active before conception and during pregnancy, unless your childbirth consultant advises otherwise.

As a general rule, your blood sugar levels will be easier to keep down if you exercise frequently. That said, it's also a good plan to carry a supply of fast-acting carbohydrate source with you at any given moment in case things go too far the other way and a hypo occurs. A great way to gain and maintain proper control over your condition is to keep a blood testing kit, sugar source and insulin injection device all in one, easy-to-reach place.

This will mean you'll always be able to test your blood and help yourself immediately if needs be. As your body's energy requirements will be increased during pregnancy, it'll be possible for your hypos to sneak up on you sometimes. Try to also keep a GlucaGen HypoKit on hand at all times, and let people know where this is stored. These are available on prescription in the UK.

How can Parents and Guardians Help?

Dealing with hypos in young children can be incredibly stressful and challenging. Raising a child can be difficult in most scenarios, but needing to work out if each tantrum is actually a hypoglycaemic episode can make things even more complex.

Teachers and other responsible adults should also have an awareness of how to spot a hypo and how best to treat one. This can include having sugar or sugary treats handy in case of emergency, along with knowing where the individual stores their blood test machine and in some cases how to use it.

Here are a few key signs you should keep an eye out for…

- Many children experience sudden changes of mood and tempor (hey, this is still a problem for many of us adults!) but if they are acting more irrational than usual it could be a sign of low blood sugar.

- Try asking your child to hold out their hand. If it shakes when they do this, this may also be a warning sign.

- In some cases this can also be combined with a 'peakier' or paler appearance.

- If these signs are present, it's safe to assume your child is experiencing a hypo. If possible, you should try to test their blood to check this, but as a general rule it's best to give them a biscuit to be safe than assume their blood sugar is fine and fail to treat their symptoms.

Examples of Sugar Sources

The sugar sources below vary in terms of effectiveness, but each can help to a certain extent. The strength of the sugar source you need will vary depending on the severity of the hypo you're experiencing, so it's best to do a blood test first.

- **GlucaGen HypoKit (Glucagon injection):** This can help someone experiencing a very severe hypo, including those who may be unconscious or simply can't help themselves. The injection contains a pure form of energy, glucagon, which can enter the system without being digested first. These can be accessed by a prescription from your GP, and should be refrigerated when they're not being used. Try to only use these as a last resort.

- **Soft drinks:** These are good sources of sugar, but fizzy drinks can hurt your throat if you need to drink them quickly.

- **GlucoTabs:** These chewable tablets each contain 4g of glucose, and can be bought from Boots and any other large pharmacy. They're generally available in small tubes which each fit 10 tablets, and which can be refilled from a larger supply. Smaller tubes cost around 80p, while larger bottles cost about £3.00.

- **GLS syrup:** This syrup is packed in foil sachets which each contain 13g of useable carbohydrate. These work more quickly than chewing a tablet and are easily carried, durable and do not expire.

- **HypoWallet:** This is a portable kit for managing hypoglycaemia, designed with diabetics and their carers in mind. Each kit will contain:

  1 x 10 pack of chewable GlucoTabs
  2 tubes of GlucoGel
  1 shot of GlucoJuice

- **GlucoJuice:** This is produced by the makers of GlucoTabs, and is a useful shot-sized sugar boost (caffeine free) designed to treat mild to moderate hypos. It comes in a robust, sealed container to allow safe travel in purses, briefcases and satchels.

- **Sugar cubes:** Not the most technologically advanced option, but easy to take all the same. Try keeping a box to hand just in case.

- **Fruit smoothies and juices:** These are surprisingly sugary, often containing just as much sugar as any cola. Just read the label! That said, it's believed they're still healthier than fizzy drinks.

Analyse your hypos

See if you can work out what exactly caused this hypo:

- Did you reduce your carbohydrate intake?

- Did you do any exercise after your meal which you hadn't factored into your calculations?

- Is it possible to avoid repeating these actions?

- Did you take too much insulin?

Carbohydrate Values in Different Foods

Food	Quantity	Carbohydrates
Boiled new potatoes with skin	40g (1 average)	5
Boiled potatoes	60g (1 average)	10
Roast potato	50g (1 small)	10
Chips	Per 50g (5 chips)	10
Mashed potatoes	60g (1 scoop) 90g (2 tablespoons)	10 15
Cooked chickpeas	90g (2-3 tablespoons)	15
Cooked dhal	2 tablespoons	15
Cooked red split lentils	80g (2 tablespoons)	15
Baked beans	120g (3 tablespoons)	20
Butter beans	105g (3 tablespoons)	20
Red kidney beans	105g (3 tablespoons)	20
Baked potato with skin	180g (1 medium)	55

What have we learned?

If you have diabetes, chances are you're going to experience low blood sugar (hypos) sooner or later, especially if you're on insulin therapy. The best you can do is try to maintain tight control by staying within the recommended limits, with the lowest blood test reading around 4.0 mmols/L. If you do have a hypo, try not to go overboard treating it. It's common to feel like you want to eat everything in sight when having a hypo, but this can easily end up giving you high blood sugar which isn't desirable either.

Moderation is the key here. If you think your blood sugar is low, try to do a blood test where possible. Feelings of tension and stress can have similar symptoms to hypos! Seek advice from a medical professional if you find you have a number of high blood test readings close together.

High blood sugar (hyperglycaemia) can be very dangerous and may lead to diabetic ketoacidosis (DKA).

Tell your trusted friends and coworkers how a hypo affects you and what they feel like, as they may need to help you if you get frustrated or confused. Both of these are potential symptoms of low blood sugar. Try to be prepared by keeping a supply of sugar in work, in the car, at school and at home. If possible, try to keep blood test machines wherever is handy also.

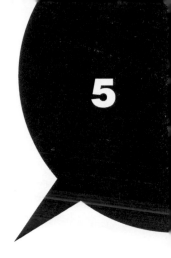

5

Diet with Diabetes

What do diabetics eat?

One common belief is that there is a 'diabetic diet' which must be followed by all people with diabetes. Importantly, there is no one 'correct' diet for people with diabetes. What there is instead is a set of guidelines to develop your own diet. When followed properly, these guidelines actually produce a diet which is incredibly healthy for everyone, not just those with diabetes.

Plenty of variation is recommended, with a special focus on foods low in fat and sugar. Following your initial diabetes diagnosis, you'll be given help by a specialist dietician who will help you choose all the foods that are healthiest for you to eat. Along with this help, you'll also benefit from learning about food on your own terms, and figuring out how your unique body will react to different foods.

Everyone will react differently to different foodstuffs, so you'll need to do a lot of blood tests initially until you have a good idea of what you can and can't eat safely.

Factfile: GI

You're likely to come across things like *low GI* bread in your local supermarket, and there's a good chance you have no idea what that is. GI has been the subject of a number of scientific studies over the past 20 years. In this time, the value of the GI has been proven by hundreds of separate clinical studies in France, Canada, Australia, Italy and the United Kingdom. Originally, the system was developed as a dietary strategy that would help those with diabetes to more effectively control their blood sugar levels.

It was initially developed by Dr. David Jenkins, a University of Toronto professor of nutrition. Entitled 'Glycaemic index of foods: a physiological basis for carbohydrate exchange', Jenkins' paper was released in March 1981. By now, the Glycaemic Index (or *GI*) is an accepted part of medical nutrition therapy in much of Europe as well as Australia and Canada. The system is now also used in the treatment of many health problems including cardiovascular disease and obesity.

Lows and Highs

One upside of diabetes is that it allows you to see far more clearly how food affects your body than someone without the condition. Gaining control over your condition can be an arduous and lengthy task as it will alter everything you do, and everything you drink or eat. For those who have only been diagnosed recently it can be particularly difficult, as this is all a new and unfamiliar territory.

Try to keep in mind that even those who have lived with diabetes for some time can struggle to maintain control every now and then, and may have to go back to basics in order to regain stability. Your blood sugar level can easily become too low or too high if your food and medication don't properly balance out. Remember that everyone experiences highs and lows unexpectedly every now and then, so don't feel bad if you find this difficult at first.

Both high and low blood sugar can be extremely dangerous in the worst case scenario, or in the best case scenario just make you feel very unwell. All you can do is keep doing blood tests as often as necessary, as this is the only real way to know if you're in control. It can also take time to get used to all of your new medications, and to find the doses that work best for you.

Both high and low blood sugar can be extremely dangerous in the worst case scenario, or in the best case scenario just make you feel very unwell. All you can do is keep doing blood tests as often as necessary, as this is the only real way to know if you're in control.

Blood Tests

- **Type 1 Diabetes:** You may need to test before each of your meals and before bedtime, as Type 1 is generally considered to be more difficult to control. This doesn't mean that it's impossible, though! (Note: You're often likely to need an injection and something to eat around each blood test.)

- **Type 2 Diabetes:** You're likely to be encouraged to blood test once a day or even as little as once a week. This doesn't mean your diet won't take some getting used to, though!

DAFNE and Counting Carbohydrates

Dose Adjustment For Normal Eating, or DAFNE, is a course for people with Type 1 diabetes which features information on counting carbohydrates. Carbohydrate counting is just one of the tools used by diabetics to work out how much insulin they'll need to take based on how many carbohydrates they're about to eat. The basic idea is that your body won't be able to process carbohydrates if insulin isn't present, so if you're about to consume more than around 20g of carbohydrates you may need to take an extra shot of insulin to allow your body to digest this snack.

This isn't an exact science, but it does provide a very good guide. We'll talk about DAFNE in greater detail later on. You'll need to work with your doctor to figure out what your initial doses and medications should be, but this can take several attempts to get right. Diabetes is a constant balancing act between food and medication.

Counting Carbohydrates: An Explanation

The information below comes from the Diabetes UK website (diabetes.org. uk), which features some great resources and tips for people who are new to carbohydrate counting. They even have some sample food labels to show you exactly what you're looking for.

If you're living with Type 1 diabetes, you might find that carbohydrate counting, or carb counting, is an effective way of managing your blood glucose levels - it means that your insulin dose can be individually matched to the amount of carbohydrate you eat and drink.

Being aware of the amount of carbs in food and drinks is important for everyone with diabetes, but carb counting is particularly helpful for those on basal-bolus insulin regimen.

Insulin-to-carbohydrate ratios vary from person to person, so you will have your own personal ratio depending on your age, weight, activity levels and how sensitive you are to insulin. Your diabetes healthcare team will help you work it out and, eventually, you may even have a different insulin to carbohydrate ratio for each meal.

Get label savvy - scrutinise the nutrition labels. Pull the food and drink out of your kitchen cupboards and find out just how much information you have to hand.

Although carb counting requires a great deal of time and effort, once mastered it can lead to better blood glucose control and greater flexibility in the times and amount of carbohydrate you eat.

To carbohydrate count successfully you will need a whole lot more information than this article. You will need to learn all about carbohydrates, learn how to adjust your insulin and be dedicated to monitoring your blood glucose levels frequently. You will also need the support of professionals either in the form of your diabetes healthcare team or one of the structured diabetes education courses available. You can find out about courses available in your area from your diabetes healthcare team.

For more information, check out **www.diabetes.org.uk/Guide-to-diabetes/ Enjoy-food**.

Guidelines also exist which explain how to match amounts of carbohydrate to doses of insulin, though these ratios vary to a massive degree between each diabetic. The amount of insulin you need to take doesn't say anything about you, everyone simply has their own unique set of needs.

For example, some people have the very simple ration of 10g carbohydrate to each unit of insulin, sometimes referred to as 'one carbohydrate exchange'. Another way of expressing this would be as an insulin:carbohydrate ratio of 1:1. So if you eat one sandwich for lunch, this is likely to contain 50g of carbohydrate, which would mean 5 units of insulin for those with a ratio of 1:1.

If your ratio turns out to be 2:2, or two units of insulin per 10g of carbohydrate, you'd take 10 units of insulin for the same sandwich. Needless to say, not everyone has such a simple ratio. In many cases, a diabetic will have a 1:1 ratio at the start of the day, but this will have changed to 2:1 by lunchtime. By the time dinner rolls around, the ratio may have changed again to 1½:1.

Some people might view all of this as fairly complex or high-end diabetes theory. Over the past few years, though, the NHS has put a great amount of effort into reinforcing the skills that come with carb-counting through a series of educational courses called DAFNE (Dose Adjustment for Normal Eating), which are held throughout the country. Websites such as UpBete also have some very helpful information on the carbohydrate content of different foods, which you can check out here: http://www.upbete.co.uk/general-advice/food-diet/carb-counting-tables.aspx.

You may find that your body digests certain foods very quickly, which can make your blood sugars rise more quickly than expected. Similarly, you're likely to come across foods your body digests more slowly to allow for a steady, gradual energy release which can be timed carefully with your insulin patterns. More information on insulin action can be found in *Chapter Three: Which Medications Can Help?*

Food Labels

When it comes to finding out what exactly is in the food you're putting in your body, food labels are a vital tool. In recent years, new food labelling guidelines have really put food contents under the spotlight in the UK. This is a result of a partnership between food manufacturers and the FSA (Food Standards Agency) to come up with one standardised set of guidelines for all food labels.

All the same, there are still a number of differences between the labelling on food from different companies, for example some choose to list carbohydrates while others only want to list sugars. Similarly, some companies only give information on nutrients per 100g of their product, meaning you'll need to do a few calculations if you're only eating 30g of something. Making food labels a clear and effective source of information has been an uphill battle and has taken a lot longer than you'd expect, but it's really starting to make a difference.

Just be careful not to only read the sugar listing when you're looking for the carbohydrate count! Check your labels and keep your eyes open: they may not be perfect, but they're still very helpful and for now they're all we've got.

The Traffic Light System

In the traffic light system, the colours red, orange and green are used to make keeping a healthy balance of sugary, salty and fatty foods easier by getting you to choose the right products for your diet. The goal is to make it easier for consumers to compare the nutritional information of these products at a glance. You can find lots of information about this system online, even through the websites of some major supermarkets such as this helpful article on the Sainsbury's website: **www.livewellforless.sainsburys.co.uk/multi-traffic-light-labelling**.

Red is for foods that are high GI, amber (or orange) is used to mark foods with moderate release sugars while green is for foods with a relatively low sugar content. Comparisons can be madeusing information either on how much of a certain nutrient is in each packet, or how much would be found in a portion of each product. You may just be surprised by how much difference there can be between two products that seem highly similar.

That said, even if some of your favourite snacks show red traffic lights, you don't need to force them out of your diet altogether! Keep in mind that not all manufacturers have started using this system yet, as it is still voluntary in the UK.

What are carbohydrates?

Chains of sugar molecules can hook together, and this forms carbohydrates. Complex carbohydrates are formed by longer chains of molecules, while the smaller chains are called simple carbohydrates. Complex carbohydrates are starches which occur in foods like cereals, pastas, rice and bread. Simple carbohydrates are used in processed sugars such as those found in honey, syrups, sugar and sweets, as well as occurring naturally in vegetables, fruits and milk products.

During digestion, carbohydrates are broken down into glucose, which raises the blood sugar level.

GI: The Glycaemic Index

In diet and diabetes alike, knowledge is most certainly power. One diet which has had a fair amount of coverage recently is the GI diet, which was initially created to help those with diabetes get a clearer picture of how what they ate affected their blood sugar levels. If your goal is to lose weight, a low GI diet can be successful as foods with low GI generally delay the feeling of hunger.

The glycaemic index, or GI, is a measure of how quickly a food's sugars enter into the bloodstream. The GI of each foodstuff is a result of a range of different factors including how long it has been cooked; the food's acidity; the kind of sugar fibre and starch the food contains and the degree to which the food is processed. It measures each food on a scale from 1-100 based on how quickly each food raises the blood glucose levels after ingestion.

This in itself does not count as a diet, but the knowledge it provides on the effects of different foods can be very useful when it comes to figuring out what you should and shouldn't be eating. The highest GI values are found in 'fast-acting' carbohydrates which break down quickly during digestion. Meanwhile, carbohydrates that break down slowly during digestion have the lowest GI values as they release glucose into the bloodstream very gradually.

Carbohydrates that break down slowly are referred to as 'good carbohydrates' and are the ones you will consume the most of when following a low GI diet. A low GI level is 56 and under, a high GI is over 70. As a general rule, any process which increases the speed at which a food will be digested and absorbed will cause a higher GI. Stable blood sugar levels over long periods of timecan often be achieved by eating complex carbohydrates such as bananas and porridge, as these have a low GI (or slow release pattern).

Losing Weight

There's a strong likelihood that if you're overweight it'll be as a result of eating too much, exercising too little, and eating the wrong foods at the wrong times throughout the day. The first step in treatment of Type 2 diabetes is weight loss, but how are you supposed to tell if you're overweight? Around 80% of Type 2 diabetics fall into the category of 'overweight'. This can be shown using the charts that are available to figure out your optimal weight according to your sex and height.

There's a strong likelihood that if you're overweight it'll be as a result of eating too much, exercising too little, and eating the wrong foods at the wrong times throughout the day.

We cannot say for certain whether weight gain is causing diabetes or diabetes is causing weight gain in these circumstances, but it is clear that they're linked and as a general rule the weight gain will be noticed before the diabetes. If you're able to work out what your ideal weight should be, you'll then be able to see whether or not you weigh more than this amount.

GL: The Glycaemic Load

A major drawback of the GI is that it only lists the values of individual foods. The vast majority of us eat food in combinations - bangers and mash, beans on toast - which combine to form one overall Glycaemic Load. All of this may sound confusing, but those with diabetes will be watching their blood sugar level, and will see clearly what effects different foods have. Adding fats to carbohydrates (like when you choose chips over boiled potatoes) makes your body take longer to absorb the food.

This is important because there's every likelihood you'll be combining high GI foods (such as jam) with fat (butter) and lower GI foods (brown bread), and the resulting energy release will be a combination of all the elements making up your meal. The GI will explain the values of bread, cheese and tomatoes. It does not explain the value of the tomato and cheese sandwich which these will combine to form, a meal containing fat, carbohydrates and protein all together.

The combination of these different foods will alter the overall GI, something which is reflected *but not explained* when we see that chips have a different GI to baked potatoes. This altered GI is one of the many reasons the way in which you cook your meal affects how healthy it is. If someone with diabetes eats a different amount or type of food than usual, GL will allow them to keep tabs on the effects their food should be having - although it's still best to take a blood test as soon as possible just to be safe.

The potential unpleasant effects of taking too much or too little insulin mean that taking a little extra time to do another blood test is well worth it.

GDA (Guideline Daily Amount)

per day	Men	Women
Calories	2,500	2,000
Carbohydrate	300g	230g
Fat	95g	70g
(of which saturates)	30g	20g
Protein	55g	45g
Sodium	2.4g	2.4g
(equivalent as salt)	6g	6g
Sugars	120g	90g

This table shows the standard Guideline Daily Amounts for men and women. A promising number of food manufacturers are now including helpful information based on this for their packaging.

For example, a label might state what percentage of your GDA of protein (for example) is contained in a portion of that food. Keep an eye out for brands, shops and foods that have these labels, as they can really cut down on the amount of calculations you need to do every day when you eat.

The What's Inside Guide

It is vital that people with diabetes and those seeking to reduce the risk of developing the condition get information about foods to help make the right choices about what to eat.

Here, Douglas Smallwood, Chief Executive of Diabetes UK, comments on a new food labelling system. Director General of the British Heart Foundation, Peter Hollins adds that '*(t)he BHF supports the FSA's approach to front of pack signpost labelling as it offers instant help to shoppers at the point of sale. We think it is important this information is provided in an easily understood, colour coded format, and from an independent source people can trust, such as the FSA.*'

The *What's Inside Guide* is another labelling system you might encounter when you buy food and drinks in the UK. It's gathered a great amount of support from a number of health organisations based in the UK, with associations like Diabetes UK vouching for how important the *What's Inside Guide* could be. Speaking for the Royal College of Physician, its President Professor Ian Gilmore states the following.

Obesity and unhealthy eating are a real and serious threat to the health of individuals and the nation. The complex nature of this threat requires a clear and coherent strategy – the Royal College of Physicians welcomes the FSA's approach to front of pack labelling as a mostnecessary and practical element of such a strategy. We are impressed by the results of consumer research undertaken by the FSA which indicated that traffic light colours are key to helping consumers make healthier choices. Traffic lights will also undoubtedly assist health professionals when providing advice about healthier lifestyles.

Some of the most famous brands in the food industry support the system, including Coca-Cola Great Britain, Kellogg's, Masterfoods, Quaker, Tate & Lyle, Walkers, Unilever, Ryvita, Nestlé, Kraft, Danone and Cadbury. This system produces labels which tell you at a glance how many sugars, saturates, salt, fat and calories you're about to consume, along with information on your GDA of each of these nutrients.

On the subject of the *What's Inside Guide*, Children's Commissioner for England (2005-2009) Professor Sir Albert Aynsley-Green said that '*(t)he Food Standard Agency's Traffic Light System delivers what consumers need: a simple method to explain what's contained in the foods they buy. This system would give shoppers more choice to make healthier purchases and has the potential to reduce obesity among our children and young people.*'

'*We hope it will be used at the forefront of initiatives to limit young people's exposure to foods that are high in fat, salt and sugar.*' It's hoped that these labels will make it much easier to plan a healthy, balanced diet by removing the guesswork from our meal plans. As Smallwood explains: '*The FSA has undertaken a long period of research and consultation to get a scheme that will be effective.*

'*However, voluntary labelling will only work if manufacturers adhere to these guidelines. Providing information in different formats is likely to be little better than giving no information at all, so it's really important that the food industry is consistent.*'

More information on this system can be found at **www.whatsinsideguide.com**.

BMI: Body Mass Index

Although not perfect, this method of figuring out the amount of body fat in adults is among the most widely accepted. The goal is to come up with an indication of someone's ideal weight in order to provide the appropriate advice about reaching and maintaining that weight. Your BMI can be calculated using the following steps. Do not use it as gospel, though: BMI measurements are not accurate in athletes and those with high muscle mass.

1. Measure your weight in kilograms (Value A).
2. Measure your height in metres and multiply this value by itself (Value B).
3. Divide Value A by Value B.
4. Check your result against your recommended BMI range.

For example, in someone who weighs 65kg and is 1.6m tall, the calculation would be:

1. 1. Value A: 65.
2. 2. Value B: 1.6 x 1.6 = 2.56.
3. 3. BMI: 65 ÷ 2.56 = 25.39.

Even if you have a healthy amount of body fat, muscle weighs more than fat and can push you into a higher BMI category than you should be. Readings will also be inaccurate for those who are breastfeeding, frail or pregnant. You may also establish if you are overweight by measuring your weight circumference. A waist circumference of over 40 inches (102cm) in men and 35 inches (88cm) in women is considered worrying, while even measurements of 37 inches (94cm) in men and 32 inches (80cm) in women can carry an increased risk.

Consider talking to your diabetes team to find out if any of your prescriptions, including insulin, might have caused you to gain weight. People who carry most of their weight around their waist (apple shape) rather than carrying weight around the upper thighs and bottom (pear shape) or all over their body are often at a higher risk of developing diabetes or heart disease. However, as a general rule, the guidelines for a healthy BMI are as follows:

- **Underweight:** BMI under 18.5
- **Healthy:** BMI between 18.5 - 25
- **Overweight:** BMI between 25 - 30
- **Obese:** BMI between 30 - 40
- **Clinically Severe Obesity (or Morbid Obesity):** BMI higher than 40 (100lbs or more over ideal body weight)

Another measurement you could do to establish if you are overweight might include your waist-hip ratio. This is the ratio of your hip circumference (at the widest point) to your waist

circumference (at your abdomen's narrowest point). As a general rule, if your waist is wider than your hips you should try to lose weight and increase your exercise. In fact, if any of the standards we've discussed here suggest that you are overweight, losing weight may well be the most important thing you can do to stop your diabetes from affecting your health too much.

That said, we must appreciate that losing weight as a person with diabetes can be very complicated. Don't let your diabetes act as a barrier to weight loss when it's such an important part of improving your health. It's often a the best idea to try eating less, rather than simply increasing your doses, to achieve a blood sugar balance. Try to focus on taking more exercise, improving your diet and taking blood tests frequently to make sure you aren't making your blood sugar level go too low.

What have we learned?

If you take your health seriously, you'll want to have a different relationship with food following your diagnosis of diabetes - though this doesn't mean your diet needs to be limited or boring! The Glycaemic Index can be a valuable tool when it comes to managing diabetes, so learn how to use it as best you can. Labels can be really important when it comes to working out how many fats, sugars and carbohydrates are in different foodstuffs, so read them!

Pay good attention, as not all labels display information in the same way. If possible, choose to buy products with clear information. Not only will this make it easier to track your carbohydrates, but over time it'll send a clear message to other companies that clear labels are a selling point. Don't eat too much, but always eat enough! Combining diabetes with eating disorders can be very dangerous.

It's highly possible for those with diabetes to develop an eating disorder as a result of the condition's complex nature and links with weight, food and depression. If you're concerned, talk to your diabetes team or check out **www.diabeticswitheatingdisorders.org.uk**. Try not to let your condition prevent you from enjoying your food: just pay attention to your body and recognise how it reacts to the different things you eat.

Unless you're in need of sugar to treat a hypo, try to avoid foods that are high in sugar or fat.

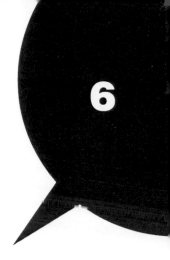

6

Pregnancy with Diabetes

This section aims to provide information for people who have previously experienced gestational diabetes (see Chapter One) and are planning another pregnancy, and people with diabetes who want to know how their condition might affect them during pregnancy.

Pregnancy with Diabetes

Thanks to our advancements in diabetes accessories and medicine, and our ever-improving understanding of the condition, the likelihood that you will experience a happy and safe pregnancy is higher than ever. With diabetes affecting around 3-4% of the UK population and more people being diagnosed each day, it makes sense that the number of people with diabetes who also experience pregnancy is also rising.

That said, as with any other pregnancy, you should only attempt to become pregnant with all of the necessary information and consideration. Even more than usual, you'll need to maintain a close control over your blood sugar levels, as these can have a massive impact on both your health and that of your baby.

Insulin

In many cases, those with Type 1 diabetes will be taking two different types of insulin every day, over around four or five injections. Most will take a short-acting insulin which lasts for up to three hours at mealtimes, as well as a long-acting one which lasts over 24 hours. In most cases you'll stay on the same type of insulin during your pregnancy, though it's highly likely that at least one of these will need to be adjusted once or twice during your pregnancy.

In most cases your body will return to its pre-pregnancy requirements after you've given birth. As we discussed previously, you'll most likely be advised to increase your daily number of blood tests - sometimes to as many as eight each day - to achieve the necessary control over your blood sugar. If you have major concerns about the potential effects your insulin might have on your unborn child, contact your supplier for detailed information.

The vast majority of insulins used in the UK have had a number of studies done on them around their effects during pregnancy. If you're currently taking drugs to reduce your blood pressure (such as ACE inhibitors) as a result of high blood pressure (hypertension) or protein in your urine (signalling renal disease), it's likely that your medical team will advise this prescription is altered to a more foetus-friendly drug prior to conception.

If you have kidney disease, this is something that should be discussed in detail with your medical team and a high-risk pregnancy specialist in order to identify any additional risks it may pose to your pregnancy. When it comes to your medical team, there are a few things you should think about:

- Are you comfortable with the childbirth consultant (obstetrician) assigned to care for you?

- How are you going to keep in touch with your medical team, should the need arise for your insulin to be changed?

- Are you comfortable with using an insulin pump if your doctor advises you to?

- Are you aware that you are likely to experience elevated blood sugar levels during pregnancy?

- Have you discussed with your team members your expectations for diabetes care during pregnancy (preferably before conception)?

It's also highly likely that cholesterol-lowering tablets like statins will need to be reassessed prior to conception. The decision to become pregnant in these circumstances (as in any circumstances) is one that should be made very carefully and with full consultation from professionals.

Breastfeeding

When you reach the point of breastfeeding (or not breastfeeding), your blood sugar levels will not negatively affect your milk or your child's development at all. Whether or not you breastfeed your child should be entirely your decision with or without diabetes, and the only issue you'll generallyface when breastfeeding as a person with diabetes is a potential impact on your own energy requirements.

It's generally advised that you continue to monitor your blood sugars closely for as long as you breastfeed, as new parenthood can be tiring enough without adding hypos into the equation. Good control over your diabetes can make these things a whole lot simpler.

Giving Birth

If you are a Type 1 diabetic, it's likely that your medical team will suggest you either have a caesarean section or be induced at around 38 weeks. This is because it's common for babies carried by someone with diabetes to be slightly larger than average, and for their placenta to progress more quickly than usual, sometimes leading to birth complications. If you want to do your own blood tests during labour, it may be possible to do this with the help of your childbirth consultant and diabetes team.

However, it's often easier to accept help from your doctor so that by the time you go into labour, your insulin and sugar solutions will likely be given to you through a drip, meaning doctors will have better control over your diabetes and you are less likely to reach extreme highs or lows in blood sugar levels.

It's generally advised that you continue to monitor your blood sugars closely for as long as you breastfeed, as new parenthood can be tiring enough without adding hypos into the equation.

Where should I look for more information?

NICE (National Institute for Health and Care Excellence) provide a good guide to diabetes and pregnancy, which you can find on their website[5]. There's also some really helpful information on the Diabetes UK website[6]. A number of manufacturers which produce diabetes medicines and equipment also have some leaflets on this topic among others (such as driving with diabetes, getting a tattoo with diabetes and being diagnosed with diabetes).

You can download these leaflets from the websites of companies like the Perinatal Institute[7], RCOG[8], Novo Nordisk and Accu-Chek.

General Advice for Good Health

- Whether you have diabetes or not, it's generally a good idea to begin taking folic acid supplements before conception if you can. Folic acid has been found to reduce an unborn child's chance of developing spina bifida, especially if it is taken from one month before conception to week 6 of the pregnancy, at the earliest. Babies born to women with diabetes often carry a higher risk of spina bifida.

- Get your eyes tested. Pregnancy has the potential to affect your entire body, including your eyes. Knowing how your eyes are before your pregnancy means you'll be able to know for sure if that changes at all.

- Take the time to talk to a dietician, especially if it's been a while since your last appointment. They'll be able to give you information on loads of helpful new ideas, like DAFNE (Dose Adjustment for Normal Eating) or carbohydrate counting. If possible, these need to be discussed before conception.

---

5 www.nice.org.uk/guidance/ng3/
6 www.diabetes.org.uk/guide-to-diabetes/life-with-diabetes/pregnancy
7 www.perinatal.nhs.uk/diabetes/projects/leaflets/leaflets.htm
8 www.rcog.org.uk/en/patients/patient-leaflets/gestational-diabetes/

What have we learned?

During your pregnancy and in the run up to it, you should work closely with your diabetes team. For information about pregnancy with diabetes, you can try contacting companies which produce medicines and equipment for the condition. Take care of yourself during and after your pregnancy. While it's important that you're careful with your diabetes at this time, it's also important you get the chance to enjoy your pregnancy.

Make sure you're wearing diabetes ID at all times in case of medical intervention, and make sure you have the necessary equipment for treating hypos and testing your blood on hand at all times.

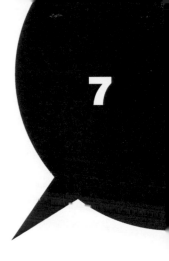

7

Diabetes in Children

I t can feel very upsetting as a parent if your child is diagnosed with diabetes. The vast majority of childhood diabetes diagnoses are of Type 1, or Insulin-Dependent diabetes. This means it'll be necessary to test their blood and give them insulin injections every day, as well as making sure they're eating a healthy diet. You'll need to take in a lot of new information, and it can be a very steep learning curve for some families, but you are not alone.

Due to factors like minimal amounts of exercise, bad diet and too much food, obese children are now being diagnosed with Type 2 diabetes as well. Your child's diagnosis will mean that a number of major and minor changes will have to be made in terms of the family's routines, diet and attitude to health. This can feel like a big responsibility, especially if your child is very young.

You will need to offer your child support and reliability for a number of years, and there's a strong chance this condition will be a major part of their life forever. Importantly, though, this diagnosis is not the end of the world.

Glossary

ACE inhibitors
Drugs used to help reduce high blood pressure, which is common in people who also have Type 2 diabetes.

Blood test machines (or meters)
Small portable devices which can be used to give you a reading of your current blood sugar level (also called blood glucose), providing a useful insight into your state of diabetes control.

Blood test strip (blood test sensors)
Used in blood test machines, this is where a drop of blood is placed when it's already inserted into a blood test machine, resulting in a blood sugar reading. The aim is to have a reading in the 'normal' range of 4.0 mmols/L to 8.0 mmols/L.

Body mass index (BMI)
This is a formula which assesses whether you are overweight, taking into account your weight and height.

Carbohydrates
An essential component of the human diet, carbohydrates are found in many, but not all, foods. Carbohydrates often include sugars which are released when the food is digested. Many diabetics calculate their insulin doses based on the amount of carbohydrates they are about to eat. This is known as carb-counting. Carbohydrates are classified as to whether they are simple or complex carbohydrates. Usually, the more 'complex' the carbohydrate is, the slower it is to release its sugars. This forms the basis of the Glycaemic Index (GI).

DAFNE
This stands for Dose Adjustment For Normal Eating and refers to an educational programme run in the UK for people with Type 1 diabetes (who regularly blood test and inject insulin). www.dafne.uk.com

Desang
An online resource run by someone with diabetes featuring kitbags for carrying diabetes kit and also a news, research and product info. www.desang.net.

DESMOND
This is another education programme. The name stands for Diabetes Education and Self Management for Ongoing and Newly Diagnosed. This is aimed at people with Type 2 diabetes, explaining the nature of diabetes and looking at medications and diet. www.desmond-project.org.uk

Diabetic ketoacidosis (DKA)
See Ketoacidosis.

Diabetes mellitus
This is the medical term for what is now known as Type 1 diabetes. The name more or less refers to having sugar in the blood. It is a result of not having any insulin in

your body, leading to high levels of blood sugars which – untreated – can in turn result in a sugar coma.

Diabetic nephropathy

Nephropathy is kidney damage. Diabetic nephropathy is kidney damage due to high blood sugars that can result from having diabetes.

Diabetic neuropathy

Diabetic neuropathy is nerve damage due to the effects of high blood sugar which you may develop due to diabetes. It most often occurs in 'the extremities' such as hands and, in particular, feet, which is why diabetics are asked to keep an eye on their feet.

Diabetic retinopathy

Diabetic retinopathy is damage to the retina at the back of the eye due to high blood sugars that can result from having diabetes. As a diabetic you are entitled to a free annual eye exam so make sure you get one.

Frozen shoulder

This is a medical condition that anyone can get, but people with diabetes have a slightly higher incidence of having the condition than the general population. A frozen shoulder is one with restricted movement.

Gestational diabetes

A form of diabetes that occurs only during pregnancy. In the majority of women who develop gestational diabetes, the condition disappears once the baby is delivered. A few patients are left still requiring medication and are therefore diabetic from that point onwards.

GlucaGen, GlucoGel, GlucoTabs, GlucoJuice, GSL syrup

These are brand names of sugar sources that can be used to treat a hypo. GlucaGen is delivered via injection and is available on prescription. The others are fast-acting doses of sugar in either gel or tablet forms.

Glycaemic Index (GI)

A measure of how much sugar is in a food and how quickly it is released when digested.

Glycaemic Load (GL)

At most meals you will eat a combination of carbohydrates, proteins, fibre and fat. The Glycaemic Load reflects this combination so is a better indication of how food will be digested than the Glycaemic Index alone, which is based on one food in isolation.

HbA1c blood test

One of the least user-friendly medical terms around, this is the medical name for a blood sugar reading that reflects your average blood sugars over the last three months. Increasingly it is being referred to as your average BG or blood glucose.

Hyperglycaemia

The state of having a high blood sugar. Makes you feel thirsty, sluggish, tired and irritable. Needs to be treated with insulin or other diabetes medications.

Hypo dogs

This is a scheme still in its early days, but dogs have been trained to literally 'smell' a hypo and can alert their diabetic owner that they are going into a hypo. This is helpful for people who have little or no hypo warnings.

Hypoglycaemia

The state of having a low blood sugar (which is the same thing as having too much insulin in your body).

Insulin

Insulin is a vital hormone which is part of a mechanism used by the body to control blood sugar levels so that, with slight variations, the levels are kept more or less stable, for example during a meal where sugars are being taken on board and digested, or during exercise where sugars (in the form of energy) are being used up. People who produce no insulin at all have diabetes mellitus (now known as Type 1 diabetes).

Short-acting or long-acting insulin – these descriptions reflect the action or release pattern of the insulin. Many patients use a combination of both to gain optimum control.

Types of insulin available:

- Analogue insulin – modern insulins that have been created to work in different ways that can fit better into some people's lives.
- Animal insulin – the original insulins were extracted from pig or cow pancreas tissue. Some are still available and some patients report that they prefer these as their release action is considered to be less harsh than the more widely available and more modern 'human' insulins.
- Human insulin – not made from humans! These are produced synthetically to emulate human insulin action.

Insulin pens

Insulin pens are one of the insulin delivery devices available. Some are made of metal, others are plastic. They can be pre-filled so insulin does not need to be loaded into them as it's already inside, or insulin cartridges can be used. Both of these types need needles to be affixed to the delivery end. Usually the insulin dose is dialled into the pen or the user counts a number of clicks, each click representing a number of insulin units being delivered. The pens are mainly produced by the insulin suppliers, with some other suppliers doing versions of pens that fit various insulin cartridges.

Insulin pump

Pumps have insulin reservoirs which are filled with just one type of insulin. They are then programmed to deliver a steady background dose of insulin (or 'basal' rate, much the same as the more familiar long-acting insulin idea) as well as doses (known as a bolus, but the same as having an injection or shot). You still need to blood test and judge your bolus and basal doses, but it's arguably more natural than five injections a day as it more closely mimics normal body processes.

Islets of Langerhans

These are in the pancreas. Within the Islets of Langerhans are the alpha and beta cells. The beta cells make insulin.

Ketoacidosis (and Ketones)

In layman's terms, this is the state of going into (or being in) a sugar coma. Ketoacidosis first presents itself as a series of very high blood sugars but will progress to disorientation, loss of co-ordination and a desperate thirst. Left untreated, the patient will lose consciousness and will need hospitalisation. If your blood sugars are high, you can test for ketones. Ketones are the by-product of protein breakdown – without insulin, the body starts to break down muscle (which is protein). The patient needs insulin, nothing else will do to address this state.

Kitbag

Also known as a diabetes wallet or diabetes carry case, this is just a bag in which you can put all your diabetes kit. Having your blood test machine, medications and a sugar source to hand in case of a hypo ought to bring you some peace of mind and might help you gain and maintain good diabetes control. After diagnosis there's no need to stop doing whatever it is that you normally do, but being organised and having all your kit with you will help.

Lancets/Lancing devices

I think most of us call them finger-prickers! A lancing device is used to get a drop of blood (usually from a finger) into a blood test machine in order to get a blood sugar reading. Sometimes referred to as a 'finger stick'.

Medical Exemption Certificate (Medex)

Thanks to the NHS, you can get your prescriptions filled for free so you do not pay for your medications. You will need a Medical Exemption Certificate to show to your pharmacist.

Medical ID

Depending on where you are, what you do and how stable your diabetes is, you may want to wear an identification (or I.D.) tag that states that you have diabetes. Some include which type of diabetes you have and your GP contact details. There are formats that take the form of necklaces, dog tags, bracelets or even credit card sizes, with some models specifically made for children.

Pituitary gland

The pituitary gland is in the brain and helps regulate the body's internal environment. It instructs the pancreas to produce and release insulin to lower the blood sugar level if it detects that it is too high. In a person with Type 1 diabetes the pituitary still works and the messenger still gets to the pancreas, but the pancreas has no insulin to release. Hence the reason Type 1 diabetics do a blood test and use the rest of their brains to figure out what doses of insulin to give themselves.

Sexual dysfunction

Erectile dysfunction (ED, or impotence) in men and female sexual arousal disorder (FSAD) in women, can be an issue with some people with diabetes. However, there are many resources available to treat symptoms, from hormone treatment to sexual aid products. Causes can be physiological or psychological and may or may not be directly related to your diabetes.

Sharps bin

Sharps are the needles, lancets and some pump accessories that are a) sharp and b) dirty (once used). Some people would include used sensors in this category too, as they have blood on them. They should be carefully disposed of in a suitable container so that no one can accidentally prick themselves. Sharps containers are available from pharmacists. You can stick one in a kitchen cupboard and use it to put all your used bits in. When full, it should to be disposed of safely. Talk to your diabetes nurse, local GP, pharmacy or hospital about this as it varies from area to area.

Statins

These are drugs used to reduce cholesterol levels deemed to be too high. Often used in the treatment of Type 2 diabetes.

Syndrome X

Syndrome X is also known as the metabolic syndrome or insulin resistance syndrome. It is currently being defined (by the International Diabetes Federation and American Heart Association) as a person having any three of the following: a high waist circumference indicating central obesity, high cholesterol, high blood sugar, high blood pressure and high blood sugar.

Thrush

Common enough anyway, thrush is an uncomfortable infection of the vagina (and other parts of the body) caused by a yeast called candida. The slightly more sugary conditions in the body of someone with diabetes can lead to an increased likelihood of developing it as the yeast finds a wet, warm, sugary environment particularly handy to thrive in. It can be treated; speak to your GP or pharmacist. Good blood sugar control will reduce the risk of reoccurrence.

Traffic light system

In this system, the traffic light colours (red, amber and green) are used to help you get the balance right by helping you to choose between products and keep a check on the high-fat, high-sugar and high-salt foods you eat.

Type 1 diabetes

People who produce no insulin at all have Type 1 (once known as IDDM or Insulin-Dependent Diabetes Mellitus). It has to be treated with insulin or the patient will die. It is no longer defined just as people who take insulin and many people with Type 2 diabetes are now treated with insulin.

Type 2 diabetes

This is when people produce their own insulin but the effectiveness of that insulin is compromised. Patients can try a range of treatments to help make what insulin they do produce more effective, including diet and weight loss. Also known as insulin resistance and previously sometimes referred to as NIDDM – Non Insulin-Dependent Diabetes Mellitus.

Help List

General resources in the UK

There are some UK companies, websites and stores that are dedicated to diabetes supplies or who have a good range of diabetes supplies as part of their overall offering. Please note that the insulin and other diabetes medication suppliers cannot under British law liaise directly with patients about their medication. However, many do have customer care lines that can offer information about actual products (not medication) they produce as well as general information on living with diabetes. Many suppliers also have leaflets – often these are available as PDFs to download from their websites.

It is possible to buy from the USA if you buy online. You'll find a far bigger array of diabetes related goods on USA websites. However, not all of them will mail items to the UK.

Abbott Diabetes Care

Abbott House, Vanwall Business Park, Vanwall Road, Maidenhead, Berks, SL6 4UD
Tel: UK: 0500 467 466
Republic of Ireland: 1800 77 66 33
www.abbottdiabetescare.co.uk
Supplies the Precision, Optium, FreeStyle, MediSense and SoftSense ranges of blood test machines.

Accu-Chek brand

www.accu-chek.co.uk
Information and advice from Roche, which produces the Accu-Chek range of blood testing equipment. They also do a gestational diabetes pack as well as a diabetes and pregnancy leaflet.

Animas brand (Johnson & Johnson; LifeScan UK)

Tel: 0800 055 6606 (Animas UK & Ireland)
www.animascorp.co.uk
Newly available in the UK, Animas (linked to Lifescan UK, which produces the OneTouch Ultra blood test machines) provides insulin pumps.

Arctic Medical Ltd

Unit 21, The Glenmore Centre, Shearway Business Park, Folkestone, Kent, CT19 4RJ
Tel: 01303 277751
www.arcticmedical.co.uk
This site includes a comprehensive selection of products for those with diabetes, particularly injection aids.

Ascensia brand

www.ascensia.co.uk
See www.bayerdiabetes.co.uk or call Bayer Healthcare (see Bayer).
The Ascensia and Contour blood test meters are from Bayer Healthcare.

Bayer Healthcare PLC (Ascensia brand)

Bayer Healthcare, Bayer House, Strawberry Hill, Newbury, Berkshire, RG14 1JA
Tel: 0845 6006030
Diabetes Care: 01635 563 000
diabetes@bayer.co.uk
www.bayer.co.uk
Supplies the Ascensia and Contour range of blood test machines.

Bayer HealthCare (Ireland)

Bayer Ltd, The Atrium, Blackthorn Road, Dublin 18
Tel: +353 1299 9313
diabetes@bayer.ie
www.bayer.ie
Supplies the Ascensia and Contour range of blood test machines.

BD Medical – Diabetes Care (Becton Dickinson UK Limited)

The Danby Building, Edmund Halley Road, Oxford Science Park, Oxford, OX4 4DQ
Tel: 01865 781 666 (customer services)
www.bdeurope.com
Suppliers of disposable syringes as well as needles for insulin pens.

The British Dietetic Association

Tel: 0121 200 8080
www.bda.uk.com
The BDA is the professional association for dietitians, but their website is well worth a visit for dietary information, with a useful section called 'food facts'.

Desang Ltd

Desang Ltd, PO Box 371, Brighton, BN1 3SQ
Tel: 0870 300 2063
www.desang.net
Supplies diabetes kitbags (bags designed specifically to carry both blood testing and insulin injecting diabetes management equipment), as well as other diabetes lifestyle accessories. Run by a diabetic.

Diabetes in Scotland

www.diabetes-scotland.org

This site focuses on children with Type 1 diabetes. Provides contact details for Scottish centres which care for children with diabetes.

Diabetes Research & Wellness Foundation

Tel: 023 92 637 808

www.drwf.org.uk

Provides lots of information about diabetes and how you can manage it. Includes an FAQ section and also provides leaflets. Visit their website to find out how you can become a network member and receive a copy of *Diabetes Wellness News*. Email enquiries through the website.

Diabetes UK

Tel: 0845 120 2960 (careline)

www.diabetes.org.uk

The UK's national diabetes charity for Type 1 and Type 2 diabetes. It fundraises for research purposes, publishes *Balance* magazine on a bi-monthly basis and provides a comprehensive website, with lots of information and a good list of books on diabetes. Diabetes UK is adding products to its online catalogue.

Diabeticshop.co.uk

Diabeticshop.co.uk, 184 Flanshaw Lane, Wakefield, WF2 9JD

Tel: 01924 239343 (order line)

www.diabeticshop.co.uk

A variety of diabetes products are available from this site. Run by a diabetic.

Eli Lilly and Company Limited

Lilly House, Priestley Road, Basingstoke, Hampshire, RG24 9NL

Tel: 01256 315000

www.lilly.co.uk

Supplies a range of insulins, including Humalog and Byetta, along with insulin delivery devices such as the Humapen.

Frio UK Ltd

PO Box 10, Haverfordwest, SA62 5YG

Tel: 01437 741700

info@friouk.com

www.friouk.com

Supplies a range of pouches designed to keep insulin cool and protected.

Insulin Dependent Diabetes Trust (IDDT)

PO Box 294, Northampton, NN1 4XS

Tel: 01604 622837

www.iddtinternational.org

This group focuses on the needs of people with diabetes who are treated with insulin, particularly those who use animal-derived insulins. The website is full of information including FAQs, facts about pregnancy and diabetes and tips for living with diabetes.

Johnson & Johnson (Lifescan and Animas brands)

See Lifescan and Animas for contact details.

www.jnj.com

Supplies the LifeScan brand of blood test machines, including the One Touch and the One Touch Ultra.

Juvenile Diabetes Research Foundation (JDRF)

Juvenile Diabetes Research Foundation Head Office, 19 Angel Gate, City Road, London, EC1V 2PT

Tel: 020 7713 2030 (general enquiries)

www.jdrf.org.uk

JDRF is the only charitable organisation in the world with the primary objective of finding the cure for Type 1 diabetes and its complications.

Kids Diabetes

www.kidsdiabetes.co.uk

This colourful website is aimed at children with diabetes. Packed with information, it covers everything – from health and the body to school and recipes. Kids can sign up for a free newsletter. As the website says, adults can use it too!

LifeScan brand

www.lifescan.co.uk

Supplies the LifeScan brand of blood test machines, including the One Touch and the One Touch Ultra. Part of Johnson and Johnson.

MedicAlert

1 Bridge Wharf, 156 Caledonian Road, London, N1 9UU

Tel: 0800 581420

info@medicalert.org.uk

www.medicalert.org.uk

MedicAlert provides a life-saving identification system for individuals with hidden medical conditions and allergies. Members wear bracelets or necklets bearing the MedicAlert symbol on the disc. Each member's emblem is engraved with the wearer's main medical condition(s) and the 24-hour emergency telephone number which accepts reverse charge calls so that their specific medical details can be obtained from anywhere in the world, if necessary.

Medical Shop (Owen Mumford)

Medical Shop, Freepost RSJB-EKYZ-SYHU, Primsdown Industrial Estate, Worcester Road, Chipping Norton, Oxon, OX20 1BR

Tel: 0800 731 6959 (customer careline)

www.medicalshop.co.uk

This site includes needles, sharps bins, impotence products, insulin pens (the Autolet range) and a choice of lancing devices, including the Unistic3 which is a single-use lancet.

Medicool

www.medicool.com

Although an American brand, several Medicool carry cases for diabetes can be bought in the UK from larger pharmacies and online from sites including that of Arctic Medical.

MediPAL

Communication House, 26 York Street, London, W1U 6PZ

Tel: 0845 603 4604

info@medipal.org.uk

www.medipal.org.uk

MediPAL is a plastic hard-wearing card, the size of a credit card that is used as an emergency ID card or an emergency contact card. The MediPAL card shows a distinctive green cross, name/DOB, emergency contact details and 10 current medications. On the reverse of the card you can list eight important medical history details (including allergies) and your GP's name, address and telephone number or hospital contact.

Medtronic Ltd

Suite 5, Building 9, Croxley Business Centre, Watford, WD18 8WW

Tel: 01923 205167

www.medtronic-diabetes.co.uk

Supplies the Medtronic range of insulin pumps and pump accessories.

Menarini Diagnostics (Glucomen brand)

Wharfdale Road, Winnersh, Wokingham, Berkshire, RG41 5RA

Tel: 0118 9444100

www.menarinidiag.co.uk

Suppliers of the Glucomen range of blood test machines.

Novo Nordisk

Tel: 0845 600 5055 (customer care centre, Monday-Friday, 8.30am to 5.30pm.)

www.novonordisk.co.uk

Supplies the Novo range of insulins, including NovoRapid, along with the Novopen range of insulin pens.

Roche Diagnostics Ltd (Accu-Chek brand)

See Accu-chek brand for contact details.

www.roche-diagnostics.com

Roche has the Accu-Chek range of blood test machines and the Accu-Chek Spirit insulin pump.

Sanofi-Aventis

One Onslow Street, Guildford, Surrey, GU1 4YS

Tel: 01483 505 515

www.sanofi-aventis.co.uk

Supplies Lantus insulin and insulin delivery pen.

Youth Health Talk

www.youthhealthtalk.org

This website is a collection of interviews with young people about their experiences of health or illness. The site aims to identify the issues, questions and problems that matter to young people, including diabetes.

GO TURBO

FOOTBALL

Tom Palmer

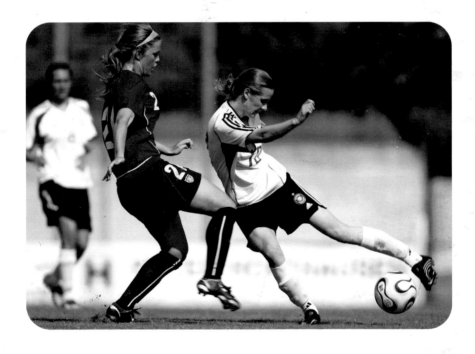

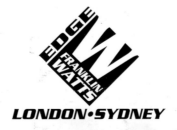

LONDON·SYDNEY

First published in 2009 by
Franklin Watts
338 Euston Road
London NW1 3BH

Franklin Watts Australia
Level 17/207 Kent Street
Sydney NSW 2000

Series editor: Adrian Cole
Art director: Jonathan Hair
Design: Blue Paw Design
Picture research: Sophie Hartley
Consultants: Fiona M. Collins and Philippa Hunt, Roehampton University

A CIP catalogue record for this book is available from the British Library.

ISBN: 978 0 7496 8661 1

Dewey Classification: 796.334

Acknowledgements:

© Catherine Ivill/AMA/Corbis: 25. © Bettmann/Corbis: 18. © Joao Luiz Bulcao/Corbis: 28-29. © Wolfgang Kumm/epa/Corbis: 19. © Srdjan Suki/epa/Corbis: 15. © Stephane Reix/For Picture/Corbis: 21. © Reuters/Corbis: 39. AFP/Getty Images: 40. Fethi Belaid/AFP/Getty Images: 26l. Pius Utomi Ekpei/AFP/Getty Images: 24. Damien Meyer/AFP/Getty Images: 17. Hoang Dinh Nam/AFP/Getty Images: 36. Anne-Christine Poujoulat/AFP/Getty Images: 8l. Antonio Scorza/AFP/Getty Images: 28b. Clive Brunskill/Allsport/Getty Images: 16. Barker/Getty Images: 22. Alexander Hassenstein/Bongarts/Getty Images: 20. Vladimir Rys/Bongarts/Getty Images: frontispiece & 14. Denis Doyle/Getty Images: 26-27. Lee Warren/Gallo Images/Getty Images: 23t. Tom Purslow/Manchester United/Getty Images: 12. Bob Thomas/Popperfoto/Getty Images: 23b, 38. Clive Rose/Getty Images: 10. Michael Steele/Getty Images 7. Bob Thomas/Getty Images: 11 & 41. McMay Steeve/ABACA/PA Photos: Cover. Martin Rickett/PA Archive/PA Photos: 13. Wang Daiwei © Fotoe/Link: 6. © Shutterstock.com/Andrew Barker: 8-9. © Shutterstock.com/Linda Bucklin: 37. © Shutterstock.com/Danny E Hooks: Endpapers.

Every attempt has been made to clear copyright. Should there be any
inadvertent omission please apply to the publisher for rectification.

Printed in China

Franklin Watts is a division of Hachette Children's Books,
an Hachette UK company.
www.hachette.co.uk